the mood repair toolkit

the mood repair toolkit

Proven Strategies to Prevent the Blues
from Turning into Depression

David A. Clark, PhD

the guilford press
New York   London

© 2014 The Guilford Press
A Division of Guilford Publications, Inc.
72 Spring Street, New York, NY 10012
www.guilford.com

Library of Congress Cataloging-in-Publication Data

Clark, David A., 1954-
    The mood repair toolkit : proven strategies to prevent the blues from turning into depression /
David A. Clark.
        pages   cm
    Includes bibliographical references and index.
    ISBN 978-1-4625-0938-6 (paperback) — ISBN 978-1-4625-1550-9 (hardcover)
    1. Depression, Mental—Treatment—Popular works.   2. Affective disorders—Treatment—
Popular works.   I. Title.
    RC537.C527 2014
    616.85′27—dc23
                                                                            2014017569

To my daughters,
Natascha Fitch and Christina Clark,
who have brought so much joy,
enriching my life immeasurably

preface

If you're familiar with the *Star Trek* movies and TV series, you know that whenever the popular character Mr. Spock expressed a glimmer of emotion, he was said to be showing his human (vs. Vulcan) side. But you don't have to be a science fiction fan to know that emotion is considered a defining feature of humanity. Philosophers, prophets, theologians, and now psychologists and psychiatrists consider emotion the "soul" of humankind. There are two sides to emotion: We are lifted up by joy and compassion, but we can become beaten down by fear, guilt, and—perhaps most of all—sadness or depression. It would be unrealistic to expect to feel nothing but positive, pleasant emotions; in fact, having this fantasy fulfilled would rob us of important functions performed by negative emotions. But some of us experience far more of the negative emotions than others. Sometimes troubled and troubling emotions take hold far too often, dragging us down into a low mood that's worse than our circumstances warrant or that keeps us stuck in the blues for much longer than feels "normal" or even tolerable. We end up losing interest in work and having difficulty making decisions. Our relationships and overall quality of life suffer. Over months and years, being ambushed by low mood relentlessly chips away at our satisfaction with life and compromises our health. If this pattern goes on for long enough, we are at risk for clinical depression.

It doesn't have to be this way. Yes, some of us are more vulnerable to dips in mood than others are. But what often leaves us defenseless against looming depression is that, for a variety of reasons, we lack the ability to repair our low moods. We don't have the resilience we need to let ordinary sadness run its course and leave us not only relatively unscathed, but also frequently wiser. We also lack the armor to fend off the weight of a blow that is far more crushing than it needs to be. *Fortunately, mood repair can be learned.* There is abundant evidence that we can manage or regulate our emotions. The study of emotion regulation is one of the hottest new research areas in the social behavioral sciences. Psychologists have made new discoveries about our ability to regulate both positive and negative emotions, and have mapped out which strategies are most or least effective in mood management.

If you feel glum much of the time, and you've tried to get yourself out of these slumps but you've failed, or you are constantly being blind-sided by a descent into the blues, this book presents 80 strategies you can use to reduce sadness or improve positive feelings of happiness and joy. These strategies are anchored in the new science of emotion regulation and cognitive behavior therapy. In the following chapters, you'll learn some fascinating facts about the nature of sadness that you can use to your advantage. You'll learn why certain mood repair or mood enhancement strategies that many people seem to apply automatically elude you, and how you can reverse that. Most of all, you'll learn specific, step-by-step methods for regulating your moods.

This book offers a toolkit you can use to keep depressed mood from dominating your daily life. I will show you how you can harness your negativity, tame your depressed mood, and unlock the emotional shackles that bind you far too often and rob you of too many productive, happy days. I'll show you how many other people have used these strategies, which are based on 30 years of my therapeutic experience as a clinical psychologist, educator, and researcher. (While these illustrations do not depict real people, they do represent common experiences and are composites of a wide selection of individuals I have counseled.) Whatever your starting point, *The Mood Repair Toolkit* can carry you forward and upward to new freedom from emotional oppression.

The 15 chapters that follow tackle the regulation of sadness from three perspectives. Chapters 1 and 15 provide brief overviews of the emotional experience we call "feeling sad," drawing on research in neuroscience and the psychology of emotion to help you understand the nature and function of negative mood. These chapters also introduce the concept of emotion regulation, the basic strategies that are most or least effective in curbing sadness or promoting happiness, and the barriers to effective sad mood repair. Chapters 2 through 13 focus on specific strategies for repairing sad mood. Some of these strategies can be used quickly when you first notice that you're slipping into a funk; others involve broader lifestyle changes that will reduce your risk for depressed mood. Finally, Chapter 14 offers a different take on improving life satisfaction: It provides six mood enhancement strategies that promote happiness and an increased sense of well-being. Meaningful change in your emotional life requires more than the absence of sadness. Rather, mood repair must be accompanied by strategies that specifically target enhancement of joy, happiness, and contentment. Sadness and joy are not merely opposite sides of the same coin, and thus work on each emotion state is required to transform your quality of life and emotional well-being.

The Resources and References sections following Chapter 15 are provided to give you further support in your mood repair and enhancement efforts. The Resources section includes lists of books, organizations, and websites that I have found helpful and that you may also wish to consult. The References section lists the books, articles, and websites that I have specifically cited in each chapter. (Some of these are cited more than once within a chapter, so you will find that some numbers are repeated in a chapter's text.)

I owe a great debt of gratitude to Chris Benton, whose guidance, expertise, and insightful analysis played a critical role in the evolution of *The Mood Repair Toolkit*, and to Kitty Moore, Senior Editor at The Guilford Press, who provided much-needed advice and encouragement over the life of this project. This is our second book project together, and I have come to greatly value the collegial relationship we've developed. I also thank Anna Brackett, Marie Sprayberry, and other members of the Guilford staff for their important contributions in bringing this project to life.

The significant contributions of numerous researchers whose work has made this book possible must be recognized: Barbara Fredrickson, Paul Gilbert, James Gross, Jutta Joormann, Christopher Martell, Kristina Neff, the late Susan Nolen-Hoeksema, Michael Otto, James Pennebaker, Zindel Segal, Martin Seligman, the late Daniel Wegner, and Jesse Wright. I also want to acknowledge several other colleagues whose work and friendship have been instrumental in forming my own perspective on distressed emotion: Jon Abramowitz, the late Brad Alford, Judith Beck, Gary Brown, Meredith Coles, the late Padmal de Silva, Robert Leahy, Christine Purdon, Jack Rachman, Adam Radomsky, John Riskind, Roz Shafran, Robert Steer, and Adrian Wells.

Over the years, I have been enriched by a long tradition of very talented and enthusiastic graduate students who have made enormous contributions to my research on anxiety and depression. However, I am especially grateful to four recent doctoral students, Brendon Guyitt, Nicola McHale, Adriana del Palacio González, and Catherine Hilchey, who worked on various mood-related projects in my lab.

I particularly want to express my deep gratitude and admiration to Aaron T. Beck, the founder of cognitive behavior therapy, who as mentor, friend, and coauthor has been a continuing inspiration and source of wisdom on understanding the mysteries of human emotion.

Most of all, I am grateful for the abiding support, expertise, and understanding of my spouse of 36 years, Nancy Nason-Clark, whose patience with my own attempts at emotion regulation has been tested on many occasions.

contents

Purchasers can download and print
select practical tools from this book
at *www.guilford.com/clark7-forms.*

1 harness your unhappiness

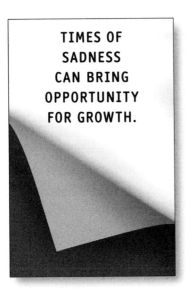

**TIMES OF
SADNESS
CAN BRING
OPPORTUNITY
FOR GROWTH.**

Feeling sad, blue, or downhearted is as natural, normal, and even *useful* to the human spirit as breathing, sleep, and nourishment are to physical well-being. But there are times when sadness and despair persist, overwhelming any sense of well-being and interfering with daily functioning.

Three Shades of Blue

Take Joan, a 66-year-old former elementary school teacher, who thought she should be living the American dream. Her three adult children had promising careers and their own families; she was contented with her 40-year marriage to Bill; and both she and Bill were in good health for their ages. They had sufficient financial security to travel and pursue other lifelong dreams. But Joan's seemingly idyllic life was ravaged by dark periods of feeling intensely down, negative, self-critical, and hopeless. These periods of being stuck in the blues could last a few hours or occasionally even several days.

Joan had coped reasonably well with several significant losses in her life. Although she had experienced two episodes of clinical depression, treatment with antidepressant medication was effective, and now that she was unfettered by work and family responsibilities, she believed life should be easy. Yet she struggled to take delight in positive feelings of joy, contentment, or interest, despite the maintenance dose of medication she'd been taking for several years. Instead, too much of her time was spent feeling gloomy, sad, and anxious. It was as if the medication took her only so far—preventing her from slipping back into clinical depression, but leaving her vulnerable to the blues on any given day.

Joan's struggle with feelings of sadness and despair had actually lasted all her life. She often woke up with a sense of dread, feeling that something awful might happen

1

that day. During these times, she was flooded with negativity and would brood about the possibility of imminent death. She had no motivation, interest, or energy, and felt as if she could cry for no good reason. She ended up doing little on these days; she would lie in bed and isolate herself from others. These frequent returns to the blues frightened Joan, because with each episode came the fear that she could be pushed over the edge—that she could plunge back into clinical depression. For Joan, living under a dark cloud also meant living in fear.

Persistent and recurring sadness knows no age boundaries. Todd was a 20-year-old university student who did well in both schoolwork and sports. He had a few good friends and a steady girlfriend. He got along reasonably well with his parents, was in good health, and had no significant financial problems. Despite admitting to having a pretty good life, he often felt down and discouraged. He had a rather negative, pessimistic outlook on life and found it hard to feel happy or contented for more than a few minutes. His friends nicknamed him "Eeyore," after the gloomy donkey character in *Winnie-the-Pooh*. Todd found it difficult to handle even the smallest criticism or setback. He was a constant complainer who could be highly critical of himself and others. And yet, despite his negativity, Todd was quite successful and was generally well liked because he worked hard and showed concern for others. When he went out drinking, Todd was a different person—relaxed, humorous, and good-natured. But most of the time Todd felt miserable, downplaying his accomplishments to himself and others. For Todd, life was anything but a bowl of cherries.

Sometimes people get stuck in the blues after experiencing a significant loss or discouragement. Sarah, a 33-year-old mother of two elementary-age children, had separated from her husband a year ago, after he disclosed an affair. At first friends and family rallied around, providing Sarah with much-needed practical and emotional support. They commented on how well she seemed to be doing, and how emotionally strong and resilient she seemed at juggling the demands of being a single mother and maintaining a high-pressure sales job. But as the months dragged on, Sarah noticed a fundamental change in her emotional makeup. She used to be a positive, optimistic, even cheerful person who truly enjoyed life. But now enjoyment and happiness seemed elusive. Generally she felt down much of the time, more serious, and more preoccupied with life's challenges than she used to be. She was more easily irritated and short-tempered, especially with the children. And at the moment, the future looked daunting and lonely. Others seemed to her to rebound fairly quickly from their losses, but Sarah was having a hard time getting back on her feet.

Joan, Todd, and Sarah illustrate three avenues into a prolonged struggle with the blues. Like Joan, many people who have experienced clinical depression are likely to suffer prolonged periods of sadness even when they are not in the midst of actual depressive episodes. Others, like Todd, seem to have a depressive personality in which seeing the negative in everything and feeling glum come quite naturally. And still other people, such as Sarah, experience a devastating loss that leaves them stuck in a persistently downcast emotional state.

Whatever their causes may be, prolonged, intense, or frequent feelings of despair, unhappiness, and gloom can have a paralyzing effect on quality of life. Sadness that drags a person down, that persists, or that constantly recurs can lead to loss of employment or reduced educational attainment, marital and family strain, reduced social relationships, and even poorer physical and mental health.[1] Those stuck in the blues experience substantial personal suffering in the form of isolation, loneliness, boredom, fatigue, and indecision. No wonder people desperately want to end their sadness and return to the land of the living.

The question you might ask is this: "How can I get a better handle on my sadness?" The answer starts with understanding how you get stuck in the blues in the first place.

Have you ever noticed that the way you feel can change quite suddenly? One moment you're feeling happy, contented, and very positive, and then all at once your feelings shift and the dark clouds seem to roll in for no obvious reason. You may be left wondering why you suddenly feel so down and blue. In fact, the cause could be almost anything—from a trivial, offhand comment a colleague just made, to a particularly hurtful incident that occurred earlier in the week. The fact is that our feelings change a lot during a typical day, and we all vacillate between feeling positive about ourselves and our lives and feeling sad or dejected. To experience positive and negative emotions is a normal, and even a necessary, part of life. However, our feelings also vary in intensity, duration, and appropriateness, and this is where the problem lies. If your sadness is deeper, more enduring, or more frequent than the circumstances seem to demand—occurring in situations that most would not find particularly discouraging —it can become a problem, causing you significant personal distress and interfering in your ability to function. At the same time, your moments of feeling happy, contented, and fulfilled may be few and far between. So the problem is not that on some occasions you feel sad, but rather the extent that your daily life is dominated by the blues.

The traditional way to address frequent, intense, and/or prolonged sadness is to ask how to reduce or eliminate depressed mood states. Psychiatrists and psychologists have taken this approach for years. But the second way is to look at how people *deal with* their negative mood states. How can sad feelings that are disabling in their intensity, their duration, or their frequency be changed into more normal, adaptive feeling states? This book presents 80 strategies for lifting yourself out of a sad or depressed mood state, so that it doesn't have a chance to get you stuck, doesn't wallop you over the head with enervating regularity, or doesn't knock you to the ground like a violent wind. *For many people, getting unstuck is a matter of learning ways to repair a negative mood before it takes hold and really drags them down.*

Some rather blessed people rarely seem sad, and when sadness does strike them, it appears to evaporate as quickly as it appears. For people like Joan, Todd, Sarah, and possibly you, however, sad mood may be a more frequent visitor, and mood repair doesn't come so easily. Fortunately, you can learn a variety of ways to repair negative mood before it digs in and overwhelms you. To learn mood repair, however, you first have to understand the nature of sadness and its function in everyday life.

> **The problem of depression can be considered a problem of failed mood repair.**

The Joy of Sadness

Human nature is composed of physiological, behavioral, emotional, and cognitive systems that interact in response to internal and external environmental demands to ensure our adaptation and survival. Emotions such as joy, sadness, fear, anger, surprise, and shame play a major role in both adaptation and functioning; they even define in large part what it means to be human. Technically, the word *emotion* refers to a very brief, momentary feeling state (e.g., joy, anger, fear), usually triggered by a particular situation and involving a distinct pattern of thinking, facial expression, and behavioral response. *Mood*, on the other hand, is a more enduring emotional state that can last for hours or even days and often involves a more complex mixture of specific emotions as well as persistent ways of thinking. *Sad mood* is a sustained period (i.e., hours or days) of unpleasant feeling. Different terms have been used to describe sad mood, including *prolonged sadness, dysphoria, depressed mood, mild depression,* or *stuck in the blues.* These terms are used somewhat interchangeably throughout this book.

> **Brief periods of sadness can be useful, helping us think through life problems.**

Emotions are adaptive, and therein lies the joy. But there can be "joy" even in longer states of sadness. Emotion researchers have discovered that individuals who are feeling low engage in more personal reflection, process information more deeply and in more detail, and may evoke more sympathy and social support from others.[2] What this means is that sadness may enable us to better accept the losses in our lives, reconsider our life goals and values, and strengthen connections with others. The title of this chapter, "Harness Your Unhappiness," is a recognition that sad feelings are necessary; but they have to be kept in check and recalibrated, so that sadness returns to its rightful place in the kaleidoscope of emotion, where it can serve useful functions. Mood repair strategies are the way to harness sad mood for these purposes.

Beginning with Basics

Let's begin by looking more closely at sad mood. This sustained period of unpleasant feeling involves diminished energy or arousal, together with the following: (1) a sense of significant loss or failure; (2) a perception of interference with the attainment of valued life goals; and (3) a belief of helplessness or reduced personal control. The mood repair strategies presented in this book target each of these core elements.

A SENSE OF LOSS OR FAILURE

A key element of persistent sadness is a sense of loss or failure. The loss or failure could involve someone or something very important in your life, such as the death of a loved one, unemployment, or major conflict with a close friend. Or it could be something less important, such as a coworker's complaining about one of your reports, a friend's making a critical comment, or your child's coming home from school with a poor grade. Even thinking back to an earlier loss or failure can trigger an episode of sadness. Derek felt intensely sad whenever he thought back to a negative work performance review he'd received a couple of weeks ago. Helen felt a wave of sadness sweep over her when she thought about her mother's recent diagnosis of breast cancer. Emily would become tearful thinking about the unkind remark her husband made to her the other night. And John felt a profound sense of sadness as he struggled with his doubts about the love of God in his life. The possibilities of loss or failure that can trigger sadness are almost endless.

   You will want to be strategic in your mood repair efforts by focusing on the chapters of this book addressing the core features of sadness that are most problematic for you, either now or when you find yourself stuck in the blues any time in the future. "Tool Finder" sections are provided throughout this book to help you tailor mood repair to your particular experience of sadness. However, don't jump ahead! Continue reading this chapter to get a complete understanding of your depressed mood.

| TOOL FINDER | You will find specific mood repair strategies that target loss and failure experiences in Chapters 3, 6, and 8. In the meantime, take a moment to consider times in the past week when you've felt down. What losses, |

failures, or disappointments have triggered your negative mood? Are there certain distressing situations that you keep thinking about over and over?

A PERCEPTION OF INTERFERENCE WITH ACHIEVEMENT OF IMPORTANT GOALS

People are most likely to feel depressed when they perceive that their attainment of cherished goals, values, and aspirations has been disrupted. Depression is rife among young adults, who often have to deal with delayed progress toward career, educational, and relationship goals. The intensity and persistence of the sadness will depend on the importance of the personal goal that is seen to be blocked. One of the most intense experiences of sadness occurs in grieving for the death of a loved one, because it involves disruption of the basic human need to be in a loving, intimate relationship with another person. Joan, mentioned at the start of this chapter, found that her periods of sadness were related to her perceived loss of two goals: her sense that she was not enjoying her retirement, because this was an important goal for her; and her belief that her friends probably viewed her as weak, insecure, and anxious, even though she wanted to give the impression of competence, independence, and resourcefulness. Carol felt depressed whenever she thought about Jason, her 18-year-old son who was charged with

> A perception of interference in the pursuit of valued life goals often triggers a low mood.

drug offenses. She'd tried so hard to offer parental support and guidance to help him get on the right path, but she felt she had failed to achieve this goal.

TOOL FINDER   Chapters 5 and 9, in particular, discuss the importance of goal-setting strategies for dealing with a perception of disrupted goal attainment when you are feeling down and depressed.

A BELIEF IN HELPLESSNESS OR REDUCED PERSONAL CONTROL

Another core element of persistent sadness is a belief in *helplessness*, or the inability to cope or adapt effectively with loss or failure. Passivity, submissiveness, and indecision are hallmarks of depression. When experiencing profound sadness, you may feel like giving up, resigning yourself to failure, deprivation, and loss. Because you lack interest, motivation, and energy, you may feel like isolating yourself, sitting back, and doing nothing. A typical thought is "Why bother? It's no use; nothing I can do will help." Sadness, then, involves a state of giving up, of surrendering to life and its circumstances. In the most extreme form, you may experience it as the desire to crawl back into bed, pull the sheets over your head, and just sleep forever.

> **TOOL FINDER**   Chapters 5 and 13 present strategies for dealing with the belief of helplessness, the withdrawal, and the avoidance that are so common in depressed mood.

Sadness: A Complex Human Experience

You have probably noticed that *sadness* as defined in this book encompasses not just emotion, but also thoughts and behavior. This multifaceted nature of depressed mood or sadness is deeply rooted in the neurophysiology of the brain. Researchers have found that sad mood involves activation of the amygdala, which is a brain region responsible for interpreting the emotional significance of sensory input. It also involves reduced activation in the dorsolateral prefrontal cortex and anterior cingulate cortex, which are higher cortical regions responsible for cognitive control, memory, reasoning, judgment, and inhibitory processing.[3] All this means that the experience of feeling sad—its intensity, duration, and quality—involves a close interplay between the lower cortical pathways implicated in emotion registration and expression (i.e., the amygdala) and the higher cortical centers involved in the regulation of emotion (i.e., the dorsolateral prefrontal cortex and anterior cingulate cortex). If you experience frequent, persistent, and intense negative mood, this most likely involves both excessive emotion generation (i.e., the amygdala) and inhibited activation of the emotion regulation pathways of the brain (i.e., the dorsolateral prefrontal cortex and anterior cingulate cortex). In other words, this book's emphasis on improving emotion regulation in order to alter your experience of both positive and negative emotion has a sound basis in the neurophysiology of emotion. What the mood repair strategies in this book are intended to achieve is more efficient and effective activation of the cortical emotion regulation pathways in the brain (i.e., the medial prefrontal cortex).

> **When you are practicing mood repair, you are retraining the cognitive, behavioral, and neural components of emotional experience.**

Sad or depressed mood is more than a neural response. Sadness also affects memory and thinking (or *cognition*) by making negative thoughts, memories, and expectations more salient, engaging, difficult to ignore or control, and believable. Behavior is affected, too: Depressed individuals often act in a passive, unassertive manner and choose to avoid difficult situations, social interactions, or effortful tasks. At this point we don't fully understand the link between the neurophysiological dysfunction of emotion regulation and the behavioral deficits in depression, but decreased activation in the prefrontal cortex may contribute to the tendency to avoid and procrastinate.

What *is* clear is that being stuck in the blues is a complex state that requires a broad approach to mood repair. You have to harness specific aspects of negative mood to restore a sense of balance and functionality to your daily experiences of feeling blue. As the Tool Finders above indicate, the following chapters contain a broad range of interventions that target different aspects of the depressive experience. In the chapters themselves, you'll find even more specific guidance about when particular strategies are most useful.

> **TOOL FINDER**   Many of the mood repair strategies, especially those in Chapters 4, 6, and 7, deal with the negative thinking that fuels depressed mood. Specific strategies in Chapters 5, 11, and 13 address the behavioral deficits often seen in prolonged states of sadness.

Feeling Sad and Blue in Everyday Life

I have stated earlier that the main goal of this book is not the traditional one of trying to help you *reduce* depressed mood. It's to show you how to *repair* naturally occurring sad states, so that they become more adaptive and contribute to generally healthy emotional well-being. To do that, you will need to know what *more adaptive* really means. What is the "natural" emotional state of the average person? What would be the optimal or "perfect" mix of daily emotion? What do most people feel on a daily basis?

The first thing to keep in mind is that there are important personality differences in the experience of emotion. Some people are more prone to negative emotion (naturally glum), while others are more likely to experience positive emotion (naturally cheerful)—and this propensity has a strong genetic basis. Therefore, you will need to take into account your own personality's constitution when you are forming goals and expectations about mood repair. The sidebar "The Science of Daily Depressed Mood" on pages 9–10 provides additional information on the nature of sadness or depression that you might find helpful in forming realistic expectations about your daily mood repair efforts.

the science of daily depressed mood

The daily emotional experience of the average person can be described as mildly positive (see Chapter 2 for discussion). Moreover, people tend to have a *positivity offset* when they are responding to low levels of input (which characterizes much of the day), but a *negativity bias* when demands or inputs become more intense.[4] Thus people seem to live much of the day in "mild satisfaction," although it is also clear that this state of mild positivity does get disrupted with brief periods of negative emotion, such as sadness. And when sadness strikes, even though briefly, more often than not any feelings of happiness vanish. Moreover, for some people the frequency and duration of daily depressed mood are greater, and the effects on daily living more profound, than might be expected. These individuals—the ones prone to protracted periods of sadness or "the blues"—will benefit most from the mood repair strategies discussed in this book, which are designed to improve a person's ability to "down-regulate" or reduce negative mood.

So how common is the struggle with persistent depressed mood? We can start with the most extreme form of depressed mood: the one called *clinical depression* or *major depression*, which every year afflicts approximately 14 million Americans, or 1 in 5 individuals over their lifetimes.[5] Although persistent sadness is one hallmark of major depression, the condition goes far beyond mere sadness and includes other persistent symptoms, such as loss of interest, poor sleep, appetite disturbance, poor concentration, lack of energy, suicidal thoughts, and the like (see Chapter 15 for more details). Other individuals struggle with *minor depression*, which involves at least 2 weeks of daily sadness or loss of interest, and possibly one other symptom such as sleep disturbance or fatigue. The lifetime prevalence for minor depression hovers around 10%.[6] Finally, certain segments of the general population may struggle more than others with depressive mood or symptoms; these include young adults, women, the elderly, those with chronic medical conditions, and individuals with a negative affect personality type. In sum, the occurrence of prolonged depressed mood or sadness is not evenly spread across the general population. The research indicates, however, that a large percentage of the population does struggle with persistent feelings of depression.

Those who experience prolonged depressed mood don't have to be convinced of its seriousness. However, there are other reasons for dealing with the problem of persistent sadness. There is evidence that people who struggle with this problem are at higher risk for developing clinical depression later, and that even minor depression can cause significant interference in daily functioning, quality of life, and physical health.[7]

At first glance, you may be surprised to learn that minor depression does not respond as well as the more severe clinical depression to the conventional treatments designed for depression. Although it is not entirely clear why this is the case, it may be that because people with minor depression have fewer symptoms that are less intense, there is less room for improvement. However, the mood repair approach operates from a different perspective, and so it has much to offer those with minor depression. The strategies discussed in this book can be used with the full range of depressive symptoms, from mild, transient episodes to more severe depressive experiences. You don't have to reach a certain threshold of depressed mood before you can use mood repair to your own advantage.

> Although mild positive emotion may be more typical, millions of people struggle with prolonged sadness or depressed mood that can be called *minor depression*. Learning better mood repair skills will be particularly important for those with subclinical or minor depression.

Mood Repair:
The New Science of Emotion Regulation

We are naturally compelled to take action to reduce, eliminate, suppress, or avoid negative emotions, as well as to maintain the positive ones. Unfortunately, our efforts in either direction may not be very effective, especially in the long run. Because the primary goal of this book is to show you how to repair sad mood, the next 12 chapters focus on negative mood repair, or strategies to down-regulate unwanted feelings. Only Chapter 14 presents strategies for mood enhancement, dealing with up-regulation of positive emotion like joy and happiness. The two are addressed separately because, as you'll learn in Chapter 14, they are not two sides of the same coin. Nevertheless, work on both types of emotional experience is critical for improved life satisfaction.

> Both types of emotion regulation—repairing sadness and enhancing happiness—are necessary to improve life satisfaction.

The term *emotion regulation* refers to processes that function to decrease, maintain, or increase aspects of emotion.[8] Emotion regulation can involve a wide range of responses—from moving to another area to begin a new job that you expect will bring more positive emotions such as pride and joy, to trying not to think about a recent conflict with your child because it gets you down. Attempts to regulate emotions can be automatic, such as when you instinctively look away from an automobile accident because it fills you with fear and sorrow for those involved. They can also be conscious, highly purposeful actions intended to change the way you feel, such as going to a comic movie with your partner to feel joyful and relaxed.

The ability to regulate emotions effectively is a key element of good mental health. Successful emotion regulation enables people to concentrate on tasks, maintain social interaction and intimacy, and establish a sense of inner comfort and well-being. By contrast, emotional disorders such as anxiety and depression can be viewed in large part as resulting from ineffective efforts at emotion regulation, or *emotion dysregulation*. Such efforts can result in an excess of negative emotion, like sadness, or a scarcity of positive feelings, like joy and happiness. Emotion dysregulation can include not knowing about or not using effective emotion regulation strategies; overrelying on maladaptive approaches; poorly timing efforts at mood regulation; or mismatching a strategy with an emotion-eliciting situation. Thus attempts at emotion regulation can be successful or unsuccessful, depending on the choice of strategy.

Ineffective Emotion Regulation

Over the years, researchers have discovered a number of emotion regulation strategies that are relatively ineffective in repairing negative moods like sadness. One of them is *situational avoidance,* or attempts to escape from or avoid situations associated with unwanted, unpleasant feelings. Actual physical avoidance is a prominent behavior associated with fear, but to avoid situations that make them sad, people may also withdraw, isolate themselves, and procrastinate. For example, you may avoid contact with a critical coworker whose complaints lower your mood, or postpone dealing with bills because you feel discouraged about your financial situation. Even though seeing other people and participating in various activities might eventually make you feel better, you may choose to avoid them as well, because everything seems to take longer and require more effort. What these behaviors add up to is that you never get around to dealing with problems, pursuing goals, or interacting with people. During her "black days," Joan would stay in bed for most of the day. Todd would end up cutting classes on days he felt depressed. In both cases, avoidance seemed the more attractive response because it took less effort; in the long term, however,

Joan and Todd felt more depressed, because their avoidance actually increased their problems of living and interfered in their quality of life. Habitual avoidance prevents an individual from coping with the life circumstances that contribute to depressed mood.

> **TOOL FINDER**   Chapters 3 and 13 focus on maladaptive situational avoidance and how to overcome it.

Excessive analysis, or *overthinking*, is another maladaptive emotion regulation strategy. Two of the most common forms of excessive analysis are *rumination* and *worry*. Many people waste time trying to evaluate their thoughts and feelings in an effort to understand why they feel so sad (i.e., rumination), or they become preoccupied with the possibility of some terrible future event and try to figure out ways to avoid it (i.e., worry). In the end, rumination and worry both only intensify negative mood. It is likely that both types of thinking are linked to activation of the hippocampus/amygdala regions, as well as to hyperactivation of certain areas of the prefrontal cortex.

> Overthinking—trying too hard to understand your problems, situation, or current emotional state—can aggravate rather than soothe negative mood.

Even though most people are aware that rumination and worry are harmful instead of helpful, they feel that these thought processes are automatic and that they have little control over them. Sarah would spend hours replaying what her husband had said to her about his affair, agonizing over the possible reasons he had cheated on her and what she might have done to contribute to his unfaithfulness. All of this thinking got her nowhere; it produced no new insights into the affair, and it only left her feeling more depressed and rejected.

> **TOOL FINDER**   Chapter 6 deals specifically with the problem of rumination in depression.

The two most fully researched maladaptive emotion regulation strategies are *thought suppression* and *emotion suppression*. As discussed in more detail in Chapter 4, our thoughts have a tremendous influence on how we feel. When sad, we tend to think about loss, failure, hopelessness, and personal inadequacy or worthlessness—so we try *not* to think about them as a way to feel less depressed or miserable. There is evidence from neuroimaging research that thought suppression is associated with increased activity in the prefrontal cortex and anterior cingulate cortex, which are brain regions involved in the cognitive regulation of emotion. You can think of thought suppression as the cognitive counterpart to situational avoidance. For example, if a salesman has had a rough day at work with lots of criticism from customers, he might try hard not to think about the day by distracting himself with other thoughts. The problem is that actively trying not to think negative, critical thoughts may paradoxically cause him to pay even closer attention to these thoughts, so he ends up thinking about them more rather than less. At the very least, deliberately attempting to suppress unwanted thoughts is an ineffective strategy that doesn't reduce sad mood. Sarah knew she should not be spending hours thinking about her ex-husband's affair, because it made her feel more miserable. But the more she told herself not to think about the affair, and the harder she tried to push the thoughts and images from her mind, the more frequent and vivid their intrusion became. In fact, the intrusion seemed so powerful that Sarah ended up wondering whether she was losing her mind.

Likewise, efforts to suppress the expression of unwanted emotions (i.e., holding back your tears and putting on a brave face), or to suppress the emotional experience itself, can make feelings of unhappiness and sadness worse.[8] Pretending to be happy when you're not is a highly counterproductive approach to emotion regulation, as Todd discovered when he tried to be more cheerful and humorous around his friends. Invariably his family and close friends could see through his act and knew that he was feeling down and blue, but pretending to be happy also seemed to deepen Todd's depression, because it highlighted the fact that he really didn't feel happy at all.

Todd learned that effective mood repair begins with acknowledging how you truly feel. That's why throughout this book, mood repair is presented within the context of genuine emotional experience. Depressed mood or sadness is always acknowledged, expressed, and then dealt with. For decades, psychologists have known that denial of genuine emotion is not an adaptive approach to emotion management.

> **Effective mood repair begins with recognizing how you truly feel.**

TOOL FINDER   Chapters 4, 7, and 8 offer more productive alternative strategies to suppression—strategies that have a better impact on depressive thoughts and feelings.

Effective Emotion Regulation

Although it's important to recognize the ineffective emotion regulation strategies you may have been using, what is essential is to learn which emotion regulation strategies effectively dampen negative mood and/or boost positive emotions like happiness. The mood management strategies described in subsequent chapters tap the many effective methods researchers have identified.

For many years, *situational exposure* and *problem solving* have been shown to be effective in reducing negative emotions like anxiety and depression, respectively. Both strategies, through which you confront the situation or problem responsible for your low mood, are the opposite of avoidance. Let's say you feel blue because of arguments with your partner. Adaptive coping would involve approaching your partner and attempting to resolve the conflict with compassion, active listening, and effective problem-solving skills. Joan would lie in bed and isolate herself on blue days, as mentioned earlier. But when she forced herself to get out of bed, get dressed for the day, and make at least one phone call to a friend, she noticed she felt better. By contrast, when she did spend half the day in bed, she felt guilty and would berate herself for being so lazy. These negative self-critical thoughts lowered her mood even further.

> **TOOL FINDER** Many mood repair skills, especially those presented in Chapters 3, 10, 11, and 13, are based on the notion that directly confronting an emotion-eliciting situation is the most effective way to manage fear and sadness.

One of the most effective strategies for reducing negative mood is a process called *cognitive reappraisal* or *cognitive restructuring*. This strategy involves changing how you evaluate a situation, in order to alter its personal or emotional significance. Cognitive reappraisal is one of the core therapeutic ingredients of a highly effective treatment for depression called *cognitive therapy,* which was originally developed by a psychiatrist at the University of Pennsylvania, Aaron T. Beck. Using cognitive reappraisal to deal with negative emotion activates the prefrontal cortex, the part of the brain involved in emotion regulation.

Elena felt quite depressed when she didn't get a job she really wanted. Even though she thought she did quite well in the interview,

> Are isolation, procrastination, and other types of avoidance typical coping responses for you? If so, try confronting the people or situations that trigger negative emotion and see how much better you feel.

she immediately jumped to conclusions like "I wasn't considered smart or talented enough for the job," "This proves I'm not very competent," and "I'll never amount to anything in this life." Blaming herself for not getting the job made her feel more and more depressed. Once she began using cognitive reappraisal, she could remind herself: "The job competition was really stiff, and the fact that I was short-listed meant that the selection committee clearly thought I was competent," "I may not have gotten the job because my skills were not a good match for what the employer needed at this time," and "I've only been job-hunting for 3 months; that's not very long in this tough employment market." Notice that cognitive reappraisal involves attributing the negative selection outcome to circumstances that are transient and changeable, and not to some permanent personal flaw or deficiency. This reappraisal of the situation won't lead to joy or happiness, but it will have the effect of dampening depressed mood. Elena began to feel less depressed when she started to embrace this more situational or circumstantial explanation for her disappointing job interview.

> **TOOL FINDER** Chapter 4 presents a detailed explanation of using cognitive reappraisal to repair sad mood. Later chapters return to this technique frequently.

Emotion expression is another adaptive emotion regulation strategy emphasized by emotion researchers.[8] This approach involves the free and genuine expression of both positive and negative emotion. This expression is not contrived, forced, or controlled, but rather a flexible, free, and appropriate outflow. Elena, for example, could be expected to express her sadness at hearing that she did not get the job. She might go through a couple of days feeling the blues, but she could harness that sadness to reflect more realistically on her situation and on what to expect when searching for a job.

Being genuine in your feelings also involves acknowledging and intentionally expressing negative thoughts. Doing this in a systematic, planned, and limited manner can help reduce negative emotion, although it is important not to get stuck in the negative thinking. During the first few months of her separation, Sarah tried to put on a brave face, working hard to hold it together around her children, family, and friends. However, she found this constant suppression of emotion draining, and it seemed to perpetuate her sadness. So she learned to let herself have crying episodes that lasted only a few minutes. If it happened around the children, she simply explained to them that "Mommy misses Daddy and is feeling sad." When she cried or expressed sadness around other family members or friends, she would talk briefly about the separation. Sarah learned that appropriate expression of her sadness seemed to have some healing effect, and she was better able to cope with her despair. Chapter 3 presents several mood repair strategies based on the healing power of planned expression.

Emotion-driven behavior—that is, behavior occurring in response to a heightened emotional experience[9]—can be adaptive or maladaptive. Examples of behaviors that are driven by and feed sad mood include becoming more sedentary and inactive, getting less sleep, being more angry and confrontational with people, eating more junk food, and passively watching more television. These seemingly soothing things may seem to be short-term solutions for feeling low, but in the long term they block mood repair.

A more helpful emotion regulation perspective is to identify your problematic coping responses and replace them with emotion-driven behavior that represents more adaptive coping. This might involve initiating a physical exercise program, getting more sleep, or learning interpersonal and assertiveness skills. Todd, for example, would withdraw from his friends and girlfriend whenever he went through a funk; he would isolate himself in his bedroom and play *World of Warcraft* for hours on end. Although at the time gaming seemed to soothe his depression by providing distraction, it also put him behind in his schoolwork and caused conflict with his girlfriend. Todd found that going to the gym with one of his friends and having a good workout proved to be a more effective mood repair strategy, because it involved physical activity, productive distraction, and social contact—all of which can diminish sadness.

> **TOOL FINDER** Chapters 5 and 12 focus specifically on learning more adaptive coping methods to alter negative mood.

Acceptance and *mindfulness* are the latest emotion regulation strategies to appear in the research literature. In many respects they should be considered *deregulation* approaches because mindfulness and acceptance make no attempt to change thoughts or feelings. The intention of mindfulness and acceptance is to allow thoughts and feelings to come and go, without any effort to exert control over them or to manipulate them in any way. Acceptance emphasizes greater awareness, openness, and acknowledgment of all emotions, without judgment or attempts to alter them.[10] Instead, you are encouraged simply to observe your thoughts and feelings—to watch them flow through your mind as you would observe the flow of water in a river.

> Adaptive coping behavior can have a "multiplier effect" on positive and negative emotions by creating conditions that activate other adaptive mood repair responses.

Mindfulness involves deliberate training of attention, in which you learn through repeated practice to gently redirect your attention away from distressing thoughts and feelings to present, momentary physical sensations of calm established through Buddhist-inspired meditation. By engaging in mindfulness practice, you learn to tolerate negative emotions, reduce avoidance and rumination, increase your acceptance of thoughts and feelings, and reduce the credibility or significance of unwanted emotions and thoughts.[10] Learning to accept one's thoughts and feelings rather than desperately trying to change them through analysis and reasoning is an important goal of this emotion regulation strategy. Acceptance became an important strategy in Sarah's mood repair toolkit. She was reminded of being alone and separated almost every moment of the day. With the help of her therapist, she learned to accept the "separation thoughts" by letting them float through her mind—not responding to them or trying to push them away, but instead passively, nonjudgmentally watching the separation thoughts pass through her conscious awareness.

> **TOOL FINDER** Chapters 7 and 11 provide more detailed explanations and present several approaches to sad and depressed mood that are based on the mindfulness and acceptance perspective.

Getting the Most from Mood Repair

The 80 mood repair and enhancement strategies presented in this book cover a wide range of emotion regulation processes and activities. Not all of the strategies will be equally effective or even appropriate for all readers. Our differing personalities, life circumstances, and past experiences make depressed mood highly unique for each of us. For example, some people are more interpersonally sensitive than others, and so their depressed moods are more often a response to perceived disapproval or rejection by others. Other people are more achievement-oriented, and so they become depressed when they experience failure or disappointment in work or career. When some people experience depressed mood, they engage in rumination, which makes the depressive experience worse; others may resort to avoidance and procrastination, refusing to deal with the problems and difficulties in their lives. Some individuals become agitated or restless when depressed, whereas others become too passive and sedentary. As you first read through all the subsequent chapters to learn about the different mood repair strategies, you will notice that I highlight which aspects of the depressive experience are targeted by each strategy. You can use this information to select those strategies that will be most relevant to your experience of depression, and in this way develop your own personalized plan for mood repair.

Joan suffered frequent bouts of depressed mood that were characterized by rumination ("What if I become clinically depressed again?") and concern about negative evaluation by others ("It would be terrible if my friends thought I was weak and incompetent"). For Joan, the mood repair strategies in Chapter 6 on rumination, Chapter 7 on mindfulness, and Chapter 11 on focused self-compassion would be most helpful. Todd, on the other hand, experienced a surge of self-critical thinking, pessimism, and hopelessness whenever he became depressed. Chapter 4 on negative thinking, Chapter 9 on hopefulness, and Chapter 14 on positive emotion or happiness would be most relevant for Todd. Sarah struggled with increased depressed mood after her marriage broke up and she had to face new challenges as a single mother. She would find the strategies described in Chapter 3 on dealing with difficult situations, Chapter 5 on behavioral strategies, and Chapter 13 on facing dreaded and difficult problems most relevant.

You will probably get the most out of this book if you read through the whole thing to become familiar with all of the mood repair and enhancement strategies. Then go back and concentrate on the chapters that are most relevant for your experience of depressed mood. At that point, do the exercises and follow the instructions for implementing mood repair during your times of depressed mood, but remember that some of these strategies will be more effective for you than others will be. You should test the strategies, determine which ones are most effective in reducing your depressed mood, and then practice those strategies so they become your natural ways to cope with negative mood. As well, you will find that many of these strategies involve lifestyle changes such as diet, sleep, and exercise, which provide longer-term benefits in the form of prevention. That is, you may find that you are less prone to bouts of sadness or depression because of making healthy lifestyle changes. So you should consider including strategies in your toolkit that have this potential for prevention, such as mindfulness meditation (Chapter 7), social connections (Chapter 10), physical exercise (Chapter 12), and positive psychology (Chapter 14). When a strategy has this preventive potential, it will be highlighted as such in the chapter.

Not only is it important to be strategic in how you implement mood repair, but it is crucial to maintain realistic expectations. Sadness is a normal part of our human emotional makeup, and so it is not possible, or even desirable, to eradicate all unhappiness from life. The goal is to reduce the intensity and duration of depressed mood states, as well as the interference with daily living they cause. The mood repair strategies are to be used for this purpose, but of course you will still have

> **The goal of mood repair is reduction but not elimination of sadness.**

bouts of sadness. The goal of mood repair is to minimize the negative impact and dominance of depression in your daily functioning and long-term well-being.

Likewise, it is important to realize that some life circumstances are more toxic than others. Dealing with the death of a loved one is much more challenging for mood repair than overcoming the distress caused by a critical comment of a friend. Finally, mood repair will be more difficult for some people than for others. If you tend to be pessimistic, negative, or self-critical by nature, you will need to be kind, patient, and compassionate toward yourself. "Rome wasn't built in a day," and replac-
ing well-used maladaptive coping responses with

> **Instigate mood repair with a strong dose of patience and kindness toward yourself.**

healthier, more effective mood repair will take time and determination. With the right strategies, however, you can learn to minimize the impact of sad mood and live the life you want.

Making Mood Repair Permanent

Even when people are aware of their feelings, they often don't pay much attention to emotion regulation in daily living. Most people are at least aware of the fluctuations between feeling happy and sad, but they do not consciously, effortfully mobilize emotion regulation to reduce sadness or promote happiness. Instead, they tend to rely on habitual ways of dealing with emotions in a somewhat automatic, thoughtless manner. The challenge of this book is to change your way of thinking about emotion manage-
ment. Rather than simply "ride out your emotions," there is much you can do to alter the way you feel. This is especially true for feelings of sadness or depression. The first step in taking a long view of mood repair is to become much more intentional about reducing unhappiness and increasing joy and contentment in your daily life.

The second step is to recognize that mood repair is a daily activity and not a single "fix-it" phenomenon. Repairing mood doesn't somehow permanently alter the propensity to get stuck in the blues. Instead, you will need to adopt mood repair as an approach to your emotional life. If I feel sad or depressed, rather than getting stuck in this unwanted state, I respond by engaging in mood repair. This involves adopting the attitude "OK, I feel sad. Now what do I need to do to get unstuck?" You can think of mood repair as a set of skills you learn and then keep applying over and over again throughout life whenever you feel sad or depressed.

The third step is to embrace lifestyle change, which is involved in many of the mood repair strategies in this book. For example, initiating a physical exercise program, changing dietary and sleep habits, taking up mindfulness meditation, being

more sociable, and practicing gratitude and compassion toward others are major changes in behavior and attitude that involve adopting a more flexible, holistic perspective on mood management. You can expect these lifestyle changes to have broader effects than simply down-regulating a single episode of sadness. They can also serve a maintenance function by creating a more positive, optimistic, and "in control" orientation to the demands of daily life.

Your resilience in dealing with life challenges and adversities can be fortified by these lifestyle changes. Experiencing more frequent and prolonged positive emotion has what some researchers call a "broadening and building" effect that will add to your resilience.[11] That is, many of these strategies will decrease the general tendency to experience negative mood, and will thereby play a preventive role in emotional adjustment. I encourage you to begin making some of these larger, more ambitious changes, because they can produce broader and deeper results in your life than simply applying specific techniques to reduce depressed feelings at a particular point in time.

Finally, I challenge you to make emotion management a higher priority in your life. Many people spend far more time and resources pursuing goals that offer much less payoff for improving quality of life than can be expected from emotion regulation. For example, many people in developed countries devote an inordinate amount of time and effort to making more money. They claim that this is necessary to provide economic security and well-being for themselves and their families. At least implicit in this frenetic work pace is the idea that greater wealth will bring more comfort, life satisfaction, and happiness. And yet there is considerable evidence that wealth generation is a weak and inefficient way to achieve greater happiness; a growing body of research indicates that increased attention to our own emotions and their regulation can yield much bigger returns in improved life satisfaction.[12] The fact is, many people spend too much time doing the things that bring them the least amount of happiness, and not nearly enough time doing the things that generate the greatest amount of happiness. You may be thinking, "I can't afford the time and effort needed to do emotion regulation work." Of course you can think this, but the real question is whether you can afford to continue ignoring your emotional life, or letting your emotions rule your everyday existence in a manner that causes ever more distress and interference in your quality of life. So I encourage you to read on and discover how you can learn to tame the blues.

2 go with the flow

> **FEELINGS ARE DYNAMIC AND EVER-CHANGING, NEVER STAGNANT OR STATIC.**

Craig walked into my office looking nervous and uncomfortable. He had trouble making eye contact and kept staring down at his slightly trembling hands. When I asked why he had come to see me, he paused, then looked up briefly and said in a faint voice, "I think I'm depressed." I asked him to elaborate on what he meant by "depressed" and how he felt when he was depressed. Over the next hour, he told me that he had always felt down and sullen, and rarely felt joy, happiness, or excitement: "I think I've always been depressed, even as a child." Throughout the day, he said, he felt either "nothing at all" or "somewhat down and blue." He added that he rarely laughed and couldn't remember the last time he'd actually had fun. Describing himself as an unhappy person who always tended to see "the dark side of things," he wondered whether people found him too negative and boring, and whether that was why they avoided him. He had only a few friends; had never had a serious intimate relationship; and, at 24, was 2 years behind on graduating from college because he had had to take breaks due to bouts of severe depression.

To Craig, his life was one long struggle with the blues. But as he continued to describe his feelings as "always" negative and his mood as "hardly ever happy," I started to wonder whether it was really true that Craig was always sad. Did he feel sad 24/7? Was his sadness always intense, or did it fluctuate? Was it possible that he had moments of more positive mood or happiness during the day, but failed to recognize them? Don't get me wrong; I never doubted that Craig was struggling with depressed mood. My question was whether Craig's sadness was as constant throughout the day as it clearly seemed to him. Was it possible that his mood state varied more than he was able to recognize?

What Are You Feeling?

Psychologists who study emotion have begun to piece together a picture of the daily emotional life of the average person. As noted in Chapter 1, we now know that people experience considerable change in their emotions throughout the day. At any given moment, they may feel happy, sad, irritable, angry, frustrated, guilty, or the like—and then quite quickly they may feel a different emotion, or the same emotion to a different degree of intensity or for a different duration. These feeling states are also highly influenced by whatever is happening around a person, as well as what the person is thinking. Moreover, people often feel mixed emotion states; for instance, a person may feel both angry and hurt when a friend makes a critical comment. Finally, emotions are influenced by the time of day, and psychologists have been able to chart a natural rhythmic flow to daily emotions (see the sidebar "The Daily Rhythm of Emotion," p. 23).

All of these changes and fluctuations throughout the day mean that it can be difficult to understand your true emotional state. Like Craig, you may feel as if you're always down, but is it possible that there is more fluctuation in your feelings than you think? Is it possible that you're not noticing times of less intense sadness, or possibly even joy? How well do you understand the ebb and flow of your daily emotions? If you've been struggling with the blues, you probably see your emotional life as dominated by long periods of sadness, discouragement, and failure. You may feel that depression is stalking you, robbing you of even momentary peace, happiness, or contentment. But how accurate is this view of your emotional life? Maybe you are experiencing more positive moments than you realize, but your expectation of negative feelings and your focus on these keep you from noticing the positive. The effect on your depressed mood will be substantial, because you'll perceive that depression is more severe and debilitating in your life than you actually experience it. Eventually, like Craig, you could fall into the trap of becoming "depressed about being depressed"—a state in which your mood keeps dropping as you become even more discouraged about your persistent depressive state.

So the consequences of having an overly negative view of your daily emotions can be profound. For example, Lisa thinks of herself as a sad, lonely, even pathetic person because she spends most of her day down in the dumps. But maybe it's really only on

> **Daily mood is never constant and static; it always fluctuates, with positive emotions more common than negative feelings.**

evenings and weekends that she feels intense sadness. By failing to recognize times of reduced sadness and even positive emotion at work, Lisa may become overly harsh, cynical, and hopeless about repairing her negative mood state. She may erroneously conclude, "There is no hope for me; there's no sense in trying." This is why doing the self-monitoring exercises presented in this chap-

the daily rhythm of emotion

In the last decade, emotion researchers have learned a great deal about the natural ebb and flow of emotions throughout the day. Several large-scale studies have repeatedly asked people how they felt the previous day or two. For example, in the Gallup–Healthway Well-Being Index, which tracks how Americans evaluate their lives on a daily basis, 54% of respondents indicated that they had experienced a lot of happiness and enjoyment without a lot of stress or worry in the previous day during the first week of July 2012.[1] Eleven percent reported the opposite, stating that they had experienced more stress and worry without a lot of happiness and enjoyment, with the remainder of the sample falling somewhere in the middle. Thus approximately 9 out of 10 Americans report feeling quite happy most of the time.

Other studies have tracked people's emotional states several times throughout the day. Laura Carstensen and colleagues at Stanford University randomly cued 184 individuals to complete ratings of their momentary feeling states five times per day for 1 week.[2] Negative emotions like sadness and guilt were much less frequent and less intense than the positive emotions of happiness and contentment.

Scott Golder and Michael Macy of Cornell University conducted a linguistic analysis of emotion words used in 509 million Twitter messages delivered by 2.4 million English-language users in 84 countries between February 2008 and January 2010.[3] This method allowed them to track hourly changes in mood across several days, since people were sending Tweets throughout the day and evening. Examining the emotional language used in the Tweets, Golder and Macy found that negative emotion was lowest in the morning and rose slightly throughout the day to peak at nighttime, whereas positive emotion had two peaks: one early in the morning and another near midnight before bedtime. Also, positive emotion was generally higher on weekends than on workdays. Negative emotion changed less than positive feelings did, and it was unrelated to positive emotion. Golder and Macy also found a sharp drop in negative feelings from the peak levels found at nighttime to the low levels in the morning, which suggests that people may be emotionally refreshed by sleep. These results are quite similar to those from an even larger study conducted on happiness words used in 4.5 billion Tweets by 63 million people over a 33-month span.[4] Average happiness was highest on Saturday, followed by Friday and then Sunday. Tuesday was associated with the lowest happiness rating. Happiness was highest early in the morning, low in the afternoon, and (contrary to the Cornell study) lowest at 10:00–11:00 P.M. A number of insights about the ebb and flow of daily emotions can be drawn from these studies:

- Positive emotions like joy and happiness are highest in the early morning and then decline gradually throughout the day, hitting their lowest point in the afternoon or possibly late evening.

- Happiness is highest on Fridays and the weekends, whereas Tuesday is the least happy day of the week.
- Overall, daily negative emotions like sadness and guilt are less frequent and intense and tend to follow a more stable, unvarying course throughout the day.
- Rarely does a person experience only negative feelings throughout the day without at least some positive emotion.
- Sadness generally follows an opposite trend to happiness: It is lowest in the morning and builds gradually throughout the day, peaking at nighttime.
- Daily positive and negative feelings are separate and distinct experiences, which means that people need to work on mood repair strategies for negative emotion and mood enhancement strategies for positive emotion.

---

ter is so important: They can lead you to develop a more realistic outlook on the extent of your depressed mood.

The knowledge you gain in this chapter from tracking the natural ebb and flow of your positive and negative feelings is a critical first step in learning to repair depressive mood. The strategies described in this chapter will be the foundation for many of the mood repair interventions discussed in subsequent chapters.

Use self-monitoring for mood repair when . . .

- it feels as if you've been depressed forever.
- you can't remember the last time you had even a moment of happiness or enjoyment.
- you're feeling "depressed about being depressed."
- you're highly focused on your negative feelings.

Know Your Daily Mood Rhythms

It is human nature to remember our most intense and prolonged experiences. So if you experience frequent, persistent, or intense depression, negative mood is what you will remember and come to expect. Over time your evaluation of your mood state will become biased, so you'll be overly focused on feeling depressed, and you'll fail to recognize the times of positive emotion. And yet, like everyone else, you probably experience changes in mood throughout the day. No doubt your mood on the weekends is more positive than during the week, and the mornings are better than the evenings.

So getting to know your daily mood rhythm is an important step in mood repair.

> Are you experiencing as much depression as you think? What is the daily rhythm of your emotions? Is there a time of day when you tend to feel best, most positive?

Rita concluded that a recent movie had made her feel sad because she became quite tearful at the end, forgetting that the rest of the movie had made her laugh often. When Jean-Paul saw his therapist after finally finishing a report for work that had caused him a lot of despair and hopelessness, he reported that he had felt depressed for the last few days; he forgot that during the same period of time he had felt happy and relaxed while playing squash with a friend and going out to lunch with a supportive colleague. Since the research indicates that there are certain times of day when people are more likely to feel happy or sad, it's important to take an objective look at what you experience from hour to hour. The first task of mood repair, then, is to collect data—to find out the true nature of your daily emotional experience and develop a more strategic approach to mood repair. If you find that you are experiencing more positive feelings than you realized, or that your negative mood is less intense at certain times of the day, you can capitalize on these natural changes in mood to improve your overall emotional state.

⫸➤ Repair Strategy ❶: Correct Your Mood Expectations and Predictions

As described above, thinking that you're depressed all the time can actually make you feel more depressed. It is likely that you *are* experiencing a lot of sadness and unhappiness throughout the day—but when you wake up expecting to live each day under a black cloud, your depressive state can only get worse.

Use Repair Strategy 1 when . . .

- you believe you're "stuck in a funk."
- you can't imagine ever having a good or positive feeling.
- you expect to feel nothing but sadness and despair.

REPAIR STRATEGY 1 INSTRUCTIONS

1. Begin this exercise by taking out a blank sheet of paper and writing down two percentages: the percentage of the average weekday you think you feel sad, and the percentage of the average weekday that you think you feel happy.

2. **Next, write down an average percentage of time on the weekend you feel sad, and a percentage of time you feel happy.** You should end up with four percentages. Craig, mentioned at the start of this chapter, predicted that he felt sad 75% of the time and happy 25% of the time during the week, but sad 90% of the time and happy only 10% of the time on weekends.

3. **Use the 10-point intensity scale presented in the Hourly Emotion Record (see Repair Strategy 2, below) to estimate the average intensity of your sad and your happy experiences (i.e., 0 = absolutely not sad/happy, 5 = moderately sad/happy, 10 = extremely sad/happy).** Set aside these predictions until after you complete the 2-week self-monitoring exercise described in Repair Strategy 2. Craig estimated that his periods of sadness were much more intense (8/10) than his less frequent moments of happiness (2/10).

4. **Now correct your predictions: After you have completed the mood self-monitoring exercise (Repair Strategy 2), take out your predictions and compare** them to the percentage of time you recorded happy and sad experiences on the Hourly Emotion Record. **Did you overestimate the amount of time you thought you would be sad, and/or underestimate the amount of time you thought you would feel happy? How accurate was your prediction about the intensity of your happiness and sadness?**

> **Do you expect more sadness and less happiness in your everyday life than you actually experience?**

If you find that you have made an inflated prediction of feeling sad, then you may be thinking about yourself and your personal circumstances as more depressing than they are in real, everyday life. This may actually be making you feel even more depressed.

You can use this exercise as a mood repair strategy by catching yourself feeling sad and then asking yourself: "Am I exaggerating my sadness and failing to recognize at least some happiness? Is my daily emotional life as negative as I am thinking?"

> **Correct your negative expectations. Does your day often go better than you expect? Developing a more accurate and balanced expectation of your daily mood can improve your mood state.**

You can then correct this bias by again examining your daily record of positive and negative mood to remind yourself what your emotional experience is really like. This way you can counter the effects of feeling "depressed about being depressed."

⟫⟫⟫→ Repair Strategy ❷ : Take Your Emotional Temperature

It is probably safe to say that none of us, at least regularly, take our "emotional temperature." We all go about our days, feeling more or less satisfied, unhappy, frustrated, joyful, contented, nervous, or anxious, without bothering to take notice of the ebb and flow of our emotions. But what we do know is that emotions change throughout the day, even for people who are quite depressed. It may be that you are experiencing more moments of at least some happiness and fewer moments of sadness than you assume. Learning the true nature of your daily mood state will help you become strategic in your mood repair efforts. You will learn which times of the day are associated with your lower periods, and which times of the day may feel more hopeful. Once you know the natural flow of your daily emotions, you can use your mood repair strategies in a more targeted and efficient manner. Thus this mood self-monitoring exercise is a basis for all the mood repair strategies discussed in this and subsequent chapters.

Use Repair Strategy 2 to . . .

- develop a more realistic understanding of your daily mood.
- discover the natural flow of your positive and negative emotion—that is, the times when you naturally feel happiness and when you tend to feel more sadness.
- determine patterns of change in your emotions—that is, find out what circumstances or activities are associated with feeling better or feeling worse.
- help you form a baseline against which you can evaluate whether adopting certain mood repair strategies actually improves how you feel throughout the day.

To develop a more accurate picture of your shifts in mood throughout the day, it is important that you keep a systematic record of your daily experience of positive and negative emotion. Ideally, this will involve tracking your hourly mood state each day for at least 2 weeks.

REPAIR STRATEGY 2 INSTRUCTIONS

1. On the hour, ask yourself, "How happy have I felt over the last hour?" and then "How sad have I felt over the last hour?" Give each of these mood states a rating from 0 to 10 to reflect the intensity of the mood state (i.e., 0 = absolutely not happy/sad; 5 = moderately happy/sad; 10 = extremely happy/sad). Thus at each hour you will have two ratings: one for how happy you've felt, and one for how sad you've felt. Enter your ratings on the Hourly Emotion Record. Part of the

Hourly Emotion Record is shown on page 29, but the complete form is available for downloading and printing at *www.guilford.com/clark7-forms*.

2. After you've monitored your moods for several days, examine the Hourly Emotion Records you have completed, and look for some patterns of change. Are you more likely to feel happy or sad at certain times of the day? In the "Notes" column, have you recorded situations that affected your mood state? Do you notice changes in the intensity of your sadness or happiness, or in how long the episodes last? All this important information can be obtained from your Hourly Emotion Records. So take the small amount of time needed to keep track of your positive and negative mood changes.

You may be tempted to skip over this exercise, because it may seem too tedious and analytical. You may be convinced it will take too much time and effort. I would encourage you to take a few seconds each hour and do mood self-monitoring. You will learn a great deal about your mood fluctuations that will come in handy when you try some of the other mood repair

> Having a more realistic understanding of your daily mood cycles will enable you to target for mood repair the times of day when you are most vulnerable to sadness or most likely to feel happy.

strategies. It will only take you about 30 seconds each hour—a total of no more than 5–10 minutes each day—to record your happy/sad mood levels. If you miss an hour, leave it blank, because it is important to capture your mood at the moment rather than try to do so from memory.

⟫⟫➡ Repair Strategy ❸: Time Your Mood Repair Work

Everyone experiences some variability in positive and negative emotions (as you'll see if you use the mood-monitoring exercise in Repair Strategy 2), so why not schedule your mood repair work to coincide with the natural rise and fall of your emotions? If your depression is quite intense, or if you've never done mood repair before, it would be better to start with times of the day when you are feeling less depressed. As the old saying goes, "Learn to walk before you run." Tackle the less depressive times of the day before you start working on the really difficult times, such as the evenings, when you may be alone, tired, and naturally inclined to feel sadder. Most people may want to start with the mornings or weekends, because that's when sadness is generally lowest and happiness is usually highest.

Hourly Emotion Record

Name: _____ Date: _____

Instructions: On the hour rate how strongly you've felt happy and then how strongly you've felt sad over the past hour using a 0–10 scale. You are free to write notes in the right column to remind yourself of any situation that might have affected your mood during that hour.

Hour	Rating of Happiness	Rating of Sadness	Optional Notes
5:00 A.M.			
6:00 A.M.			
7:00 A.M.			
8:00 A.M.			
9:00 A.M.			
10:00 A.M.			

Use Repair Strategy 3 when . . .

- there are regular times of the day that are most difficult—that is, when you feel most depressed.
- there are regular times of the day when your mood is more positive.
- your depression is intense and less responsive to mood repair.
- intentional mood repair is new to you.

REPAIR STRATEGY 3 INSTRUCTIONS

1. Since the mornings are least often associated with sad mood, start working on any negative mood you might experience in the morning. Why not take advantage of the natural flow of daily emotion?

2. Once you've had some success with repairing sadness in the morning, focus on the afternoon, when dysphoria is more likely and possibly even more intense.

Dealing with depressed mood in the afternoon may be more difficult, because that's the time of day most often associated with negative mood and stress.

Craig discovered from his Hourly Emotion Records that he felt low or sad a far greater percentage of the day than the average person. However, like others, he had more times of feeling slightly more positive and less depressed from 10:00 a.m. to 12:00 noon. He still rated himself higher in sadness than in happiness, but the difference between the two ratings was not as great during late morning as it was in late afternoon and early evening. Given the importance of having some success with mood repair at the beginning, Craig used some of the cognitive and behavioral mood repair strategies presented in subsequent chapters to repair his negative mood in late morning. After some success with this time interval, he was ready to tackle the bigger problem of depressed mood in late afternoon, as well as on Friday and Saturday evenings.

> Timing your mood repair will be an important strategy you'll want to use with all the other mood repair interventions. Consider bookmarking this page and returning to it frequently, to remind yourself to be strategic in the timing of your mood repair efforts.

⧉⧉⧉➡ Repair Strategy ❹: Create a Mood Hierarchy

Over the decades, psychologists have discovered two fundamental interventions that have proven highly successful in treating clinical anxiety and depression. The first is breaking down a complicated problem into its component parts and then working on each component in a systematic fashion. The second approach, originally introduced in the treatment of anxiety, is the development of an *exposure hierarchy*—a list of feared situations, ranked from least to most feared. The anxious person is first exposed to a mildly feared situation; once that is conquered, the individual moves up the hierarchy to the next most feared situation, until the most intensely frightening situation at the top of the hierarchy is conquered. The same approach can be used to schedule your mood repair work.

Use Repair Strategy 4 when . . .

- you are feeling overwhelmed by depression.
- you are feeling "depressed about being depressed."
- you haven't experienced much success with improving depressed mood.
- you are new to mood repair.

REPAIR STRATEGY 4 INSTRUCTIONS

1. Go back over your Hourly Emotion Records, and note times throughout the day when you have varying levels of sad mood. For example, there may be certain times or situations in which negative mood is fairly mild (1–3), other times when it is moderate (4–6), and still other times when it is fairly intense (7–10).

2. You should also have recorded some situations in the "Notes" column that are associated with varying intensities of sadness. Rank these times and situations from least to most depressing.

3. Use these rankings to guide you in constructing a mood repair schedule. Start near the bottom of the hierarchy, and work your way up to the times/situations associated with the most intense negative mood.

Although the notion of a *mood hierarchy* is not commonly used in the treatment of depression, there is reason to believe that it could be helpful, given the evidence for the hierarchy approach's effectiveness in treating fear and anxiety disorders (another group of emotional disturbances). It makes sense to start with mood repair during times of the day when you are less depressed, and then, once you've succeeded in improving your mood during those times, to move on to the moderately intense and then more extreme times of feeling blue. For most people, times when they are alone are more depressing than times when they are interacting with others, such as at work or recreation. Thus times when you are alone might be placed toward the top of your mood hierarchy. You would not start mood repair at such a time, but rather when you have briefer, less intense sadness—when, let's say, you are driving to work. That time of the day might be lower on your mood hierarchy because the sadness is briefer and less intense.

> Be strategic; focus on times when your sadness is less intense, and then work up to your worst times of the day.

The Importance of Being Earnest: Commit Yourself to Mood Monitoring

Many of us tend to view our emotions as beyond our control—as biological responses to life situations that lie outside the influence of corrective, intentional thought. Research on emotion has shown that we have much greater ability to regulate our emotional life than we might previously have thought possible. Effective emotion regulation does, however, require a more accurate understanding of our emotions, as well as a systematic, intentional approach to emotion management. Negative mood repair plays a key role in emotion regulation. To improve your mood repair skills, it is critical to have an accurate understanding of your daily mood state. This will only be possible if you obtain a baseline assessment of the frequency and intensity of your positive and negative mood states, as well as the circumstances associated with changes in these states.

The strategies presented in this chapter all focus on monitoring your daily mood states. The information you will obtain from these exercises will be critical to using the cognitive and behavioral mood repair strategies discussed in subsequent chapters. As a bonus, you may find that simply monitoring your daily moods will actually change your emotional well-being for the better. Psychologists have known for years that just keeping track of certain thoughts, feelings, or behaviors can have a significant effect on our experience.

Many years ago, I was working with people on the waiting list for participation in one of the first clinical trials of cognitive behavior therapy for panic disorder. The patients simply recorded information on their panic attacks in a daily log; there was no active treatment. However, my colleagues and I noted that after 3–4 weeks these waiting-list patients actually experienced a decline in their panic attacks, although it was not as great as for the individuals receiving treatment. We think that by systematically tracking their panic attacks, people learned that the attacks were not as bad as they had thought. The same positive effect could happen to you once you begin using the Hourly Emotion Record: You will gain a greater understanding of the daily changes in your feelings of sadness and happiness, and this new insight may itself have a positive effect on your daily mood states.

> Simply monitoring the fluctuations and changes in your daily mood can have a positive mood-altering effect in its own right.

I hope you will begin your mood repair program with the monitoring exercises described in this chapter. By earnestly committing yourself to a brief period of systematic, conscientious mood monitoring, you will be well positioned to start correcting the imbalances in your emotional experience.

3 trap your "tigers"

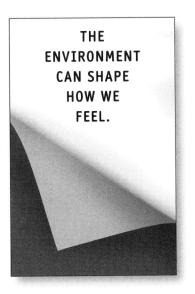

THE ENVIRONMENT CAN SHAPE HOW WE FEEL.

By his late 20s, Hector had already struggled with recurring bouts of depression for several years. Over the last few months, his depressive mood episodes had become more frequent and intense—largely due to many life difficulties and disappointments that were stifling his independence and maturity. He was forced to drop out of the university before getting his degree because of overwhelming fatigue and poor performance. He tried to work at a series of low-paying jobs, but the best he could do was hold down a part-time job delivering pizza. Lacking financial resources, he had to move back home and live with his aging parents in a rural part of the state. He had practically no contact with the few friends he had made at school. After his long-time girlfriend broke up with him, Hector had avoided dating for the last 2 years and was now watching his friends surpass him in establishing careers and families. He also had a chronic skin condition and a weight problem, both of which embarrassed him and made him withdraw. Hector often thought to himself how much his life "sucked." His experiences of loss and failure seemed inevitable; they were like "tigers" lurking in the jungle, ready to pounce on him and devour his very existence. Around every corner, there seemed to be a new failure or disappointment just waiting for him. Whenever he thought about his life or pondered his circumstances, he felt more and more depressed. For Hector, there seemed no way out of his current misery and despair.

For many people, life's problems, situations, and circumstances are a major cause of their inability to shake the blues. Disrupted relationships, financial burdens, health problems, educational or career failures, child-related issues, and inadequate housing are just a few of the numerous ways life can drag people down. You may be feeling that one bad thing after another has happened to you, and you are waiting for the next big disappointment in your life. You might be feeling like hunted prey, with fate acting like a tiger that is stalking you, looking to exploit your weakest moment.

Use the strategies in this chapter particularly if . . .

- you are feeling ambushed by life's unexpected twists and turns, or depressed by your "impossible circumstances."
- you've experienced significant losses and failures in your life.
- you feel overwhelmed by daily stresses and demands at home or work.
- you feel as if you're falling behind, unable to deal with personal problems.
- it seems that your life is out of control and you are a victim of circumstances.

Life's "Tigers": The Triggers of Sadness

I've never hunted tigers. I've seen tiger hunts on movies and documentaries, but my personal experience is limited to our house cat, April, who thought she was a tiger when hunting for mice. What I observed was her incredible patience—lying in wait if she thought she had cornered a mouse, waiting for the opportune moment to pounce on her prey. People who get stuck in the blues often feel as if life is filled with tigers lying in wait for them. Of course, the challenges and difficulties of life aren't lying in wait for you, although it is true that the events and circumstances of daily life have a huge impact on mood and that everyone has to deal with unexpected turns of events. If you've been feeling more like the mouse than the cat—with life problems and circumstances seeming to spring on you from nowhere, leaving you weakened, vulnerable, and depressed—it's time to turn the tables and start hunting for tigers.

What happens throughout the day has a major impact on how we feel. Our life circumstances, the situations we find ourselves in, how people treat us and react to us—all of these things contribute to our feeling positive or negative. You may be feeling depressed because of a major life event (such as the death of a loved one or unemployment), or the accumulation of much smaller problems (like a long, frustrating commute to work or an old house that needs constant small repairs). Even minor changes in the physical environment can affect mood. For example, sitting in a cramped, hot, and stuffy room will cause negative feelings in most people.

Research that has tracked changes in people's daily mood has found that even minor stressors have a significant impact on mood, with interpersonal conflicts or tensions causing the greatest fluctuations. In one study of working women, certain daily activities such as work pressures and commuting were associated with lower happiness, whereas shopping and relaxing with friends were related to higher happiness ratings.[1] Thus it is important to ask yourself: "What is happening in my life right now that might be making me feel sad and discouraged?"

> Searching for "tigers," which
> are the daily external problems,
> stressors, and demands that
> trigger your depressed mood, is
> an important part of mood repair.

As discussed in Chapter 1, events and situations that involve a sense of personal loss or failure, that are perceived as disrupting valued personal goals, or that leave you thinking you are helpless and unable to control the outcome are those most likely to trigger negative emotion. But another element can increase the likelihood that sad mood will take hold: your reaction to these events and situations. If you actually believe that life is full of tigers that are out to get you, you may be more vulnerable to their negative impact. If, for example, you interpret a criticism by your boss as a sign that she doesn't like you and is likely to fire you, your mood will plummet, whereas viewing this as an isolated comment that you can address may quickly repair your disappointment and allow you to avoid getting stuck in the blues. The mood repair strategies in this chapter focus on the external triggers, the tigers in your life, that cause periods of sadness. Dealing with these triggers is an important type of mood repair. To make these strategies work for you, you will be asking yourself two key questions:

- *What are my tigers?* What has happened today that involves apparent loss, failure, helplessness, or disruption of my goals, and thus might be triggering my depressed mood?
- *What is my response?* How am I thinking about this situation, evaluating it, or interpreting it that is making me feel depressed? How am I trying to deal with it?

⟫⟫➡ Repair Strategy ❺: Hunt Your Tigers by Using Situation Monitoring

The external triggers of depressed mood can be like tigers hiding in the grass: You may hardly be aware of their effect on your mood because you're unaware of them or you've become used to them. Or maybe you don't fully appreciate their negative effect; you know these problems exist, but you underestimate their negative impact on you. Or you may be very aware of your depressed feelings, but what is causing them may not be nearly so obvious. And some external triggers can simply be subtle and transitory. It can be easy to be aware that a fight with your spouse or a poor performance review at work got you down, but much harder to see that a scratch on a new piece of furniture or an unkind comment by a close friend really got to you. Also, a trigger may not have occurred just now, but instead may be caused by thinking back to a past negative event. You might also be thinking that the event should not be bothering you, and so you try to deny or rationalize its effect. All of these factors mean that identifying the external situations and circumstances associated with feeling depressed may be a difficult task.

> **The longer we live with a difficult situation, the harder it can be to fully appreciate its negative personal impact. Our problems can remain partially or completely hidden to us, like tigers that are hiding in the grass.**

Use Repair Strategy 5 when . . .

- you don't know why you feel depressed so often.
- your sadness seems to appear "out of the blue" for no apparent reason.
- you're not sure how much your daily life situation affects your mood state.

REPAIR STRATEGY 5 INSTRUCTIONS

The following are a few steps you can take to identify the unrecognized triggers of your sadness.

1. **Go back over the mood monitoring you did earlier (see Chapter 2), and notice some of the negative things that happened around the time you were feeling down.** What was happening in your life, or what were you thinking that involved loss, failure, disappointment, or helplessness? Who were you with, what were you doing, and where did it happen? What bothered you about this situation? Which events were associated with an increase in positive mood, and which were associated with an increase in negative or depressed mood?

2. **Over the next week or two, do some more mood monitoring, but this time complete this sentence: "I am feeling depressed right now because** _____."

3. **Look for particular themes or trends in the situations associated with your episodes of negative feelings. Be on the lookout for events or situations that tend to repeat themselves from one day to the next.** These repetitive events may play a significant role in driving you further into the blues. For example, if people's opinions are very important to you, an unkind remark or not being included may be experiences that you find particularly depressing. If you are a perfectionist, making mistakes or failing to meet a high standard of competence may be most depressing. Whatever it is, look for some heightened sensitivity to certain kinds of events that trigger depressed mood.

4. **If you did not record triggering situations on the Hourly Emotion Record (see Repair Strategy 2 in Chapter 2), complete the Hourly Emotion Record again for 2 weeks, but this time focus on what is happening to you each hour of the day that might be affecting your mood state.** Which events are associated with an increase in positive mood, and which with an increase in negative mood? Does each event or circumstance have a strong or weak effect on your mood state?

5. **Note whether during times of more intense sadness you are thinking back to a significant major life event, such as some interpersonal or family conflict, financial loss, a medical condition, or the like.** Are you spending a lot of time thinking about this stressful situation, and is this triggering bouts of depressed mood? Recalling past losses and failures can have a profound impact on your mood.

> **Hunt for everyday situations involving perceived loss, failure, or disappointment that may trigger recurring bouts of negative mood.**

This exercise is the basis of all the other mood repair strategies in this chapter. You need to identify repetitive situations that tend to have a significant effect on your depressed mood—and also unique ones that are happening only in this moment—before you can deal with these triggers and reduce your sadness.

➤➤➤ Repair Strategy ❻: Cage Your Tigers by Minimizing Negative Effects

If we continue with the tiger analogy, one obvious way to improve your mood state is to see whether you can cage your tigers—that is, whether you can contain or minimize the negative impact of your life problems, situations, or circumstances on your emotional well-being. Marilyn noticed that she always felt worse after a telephone conversation with her mother-in-law, because it seemed as if there was nothing she could do right. Her mother-in-law was critical of her housecleaning routine, her parenting practices, and the way she related to her husband. There was nothing that Marilyn could do to earn a positive comment from her mother-in-law. So she decided that she needed to limit the calls to once weekly. Mike, her husband, also agreed to answer the phone when his mother called. Although Marilyn could not completely avoid her mother-in-law, she was able to limit a source of negativity in her life; she was able, to some extent, to cage this particular tiger. Once you've completed the situation-monitoring exercise described above and have identified the triggers of your depressed mood, you can use this exercise to determine how to reduce their negative effects on you.

Use Repair Strategy 6 when . . .

- there is a specific person or situation that consistently leads to a worsening of your depressed mood.
- you're not constantly preoccupied with thinking about the person or situation.
- it is possible to reduce contact with the person or situation without undue interference or inconvenience in your life.

REPAIR STRATEGY 6 INSTRUCTIONS

1. **Determine whether you can reduce your exposure to difficult or negative people/situations.** It may be that you've been living with a difficult problem or situation for a long time. Reexamine the depressive situation from the perspective of reducing your exposure to it, or at least minimizing its negative effects on your mood. Let's say, for example, that one of your coworkers is a particularly negative individual who is always complaining about others. In doing your situation-monitoring work, you notice that being around this coworker brings down your mood state. Can you think of ways to avoid (or at least reduce the amount of time you spend with) this person? Or if going to the bar and having a few drinks makes you feel more depressed, then work on reducing this type of behavior. If you notice that watching too much television or getting into arguments with your spouse/partner is associated with negative mood, then reductions in both types of behavior may be the key to improving this mood. Sometimes you can't resolve a depressing situation or completely avoid a person who gets you down, but you can look for ways to reduce the negative impact on your emotional state.

2. **After reducing exposure to this difficult situation or person, evaluate whether this has resulted in a direct improvement in your mood *without* causing undue interference or distress in your daily life.** It is important that your efforts to minimize the negative impact of triggers to depressed mood do not turn into chronic avoidance. As we will see in Chapter 13, procrastination and other forms of avoidance can actually increase depressed mood. So constantly avoiding a difficult spouse, procrastinating on a challenging project, or failing to follow up on a friend's invitation are not minimization or avoidance responses that promote mood repair. In the long term, these responses will lead to greater unhappiness because of the

> Minimizing contact with a negative person or situation can be a useful mood repair strategy, provided that it does not lead to long-term avoidance and procrastination.

negative consequences the avoidance creates. When reducing exposure to a difficult person or situation, you must make sure you are not simply avoiding a problem that could be dealt with more effectively by the problem-solving strategy discussed at the end of this chapter (see Repair Strategy 10).

Hector identified many aspects of his current life situation that lowered his mood. Working at a low-paying part-time job, living with his parents, failing to complete school, and not having dated for 2 years were just some of the triggers for his daily depressed mood episodes. He decided that the problem of living at home could be improved if he reduced the amount of time he spent with his parents in the evening. His mother, in particular, bothered him with her constant advice on how he could meet young women, while his father complained about finances and how hard it was to live on a fixed retirement income. Hector worked on scheduling various activities for the evening that might get him out of the house. Sometimes minimizing contact with a depressing person or situation is one of the best mood repair strategies.

3. *Minimize* **negativity; don't try to eliminate it.** I should add a caveat at this point: I am not talking about eliminating all negativity in your life, as preached by many of society's popular positive thinking and motivational gurus. Barbara Ehrenreich, in her book *Bright-Sided: How the Relentless Promotion of Positive Thinking Has Undermined America* (released in the U.K. as *Smile or Die: How Positive Thinking Fooled America and the World*), makes a persuasive argument that negative information and criticism can be helpful and should not be avoided or dismissed in order to preserve an unrealistic and biased positive outlook. After all, you wouldn't want to ignore a hurricane warning issued to your community because it was too negative. What I am advocating is to minimize a barrage of negativity that is having a significant influence on your general emotional state.

➤➤➤ Repair Strategy ❼: Take Charge of the Hunt with a Responsibility Chart

The majority of life circumstances that make you feel down may not be controllable through minimization or avoidance. In these cases, the only solution may be to change the situation. To continue with the tiger metaphor, you may need to "take charge of the hunt"—that is, to take responsibility for unpleasant circumstances by changing how you deal with them. But before you can do this, it is important to have a realistic understanding of the level of personal control and responsibility you have over each event. If you overestimate your control and responsibility, you will be frustrated by your attempts to change the situation, and you may end up feeling even more depressed. So the first thing to do before creating an action plan is to arrive at a realistic appraisal of your responsibility and control. The responsibility chart shown below is a useful tool for this purpose. The circle or "pie" represents the totality of factors that might be responsible for a particular problem. The idea is to divide the pie into sections, with each section representing the percentage of control or responsibility a factor might have in creating the problem. The percentages must add up to 100%.

Use Repair Strategy 7 when . . .

- you have a tendency to assume too much responsibility for negative things that happen to your family, at work, or in the neighborhood.
- you often feel powerless to make changes in difficult personal circumstances.
- difficult situations or people don't change, despite your best efforts.

REPAIR STRATEGY 7 INSTRUCTIONS

1. Write a list of all the factors that might contribute to a problem (other people, external factors, timing, your own behavior, etc.).

SAMPLE RESPONSIBILITY CHART

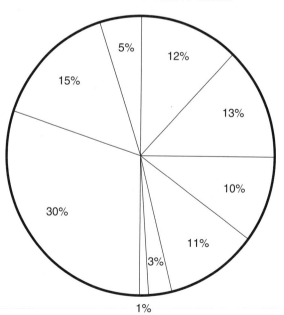

2. Next, try to rank these factors from the most influential (the ones contributing the most to the problem) to the least influential.

3. Now assign a percentage of responsibility/control to each factor.

4. Look at the percentage of personal responsibility or control you have over the situation.

5. **Reflect on whether you have assumed you had more responsibility or control over the situation than is realistic.** If you are overestimating your personal control, it is important to scale back your efforts to change the situation. Reevaluate just how much difference you can make in the situation, given the levels of responsibility/control represented in the responsibility chart.

Realizing that you have much less control and responsibility over changing a negative situation than you may have thought can in itself improve your mood state, because now you can work on accepting the things that you cannot change and limiting your efforts to aspects of the problem that are under your control. This sentiment may be best summed up in the well-known Serenity Prayer used in many Twelve-Step organizations, such as Alcoholics Anonymous:

> God, grant me the serenity to accept the things I cannot change,
> The courage to change the things I can,
> And wisdom to know the difference.

Hector worked on a responsibility chart for his chronic skin problem. For years he had felt depressed and discouraged by flare-ups of this embarrassing skin rash, which seemed to happen at the most inopportune times. He'd tried numerous creams, medications, and other strategies to control the skin rash, but to no avail. After completing the responsibility chart (see the next page), Hector realized that he had much less control over the skin rash (i.e., 6%) than he had assumed. Some of the biggest contributors, such as genetics and the environment, were entirely outside his control. What Hector realized was that he needed to abandon his control efforts and work on accepting the skin condition.

⤷⤷⤷ Repair Strategy ⑧: Face the Tiger through Expressive Writing

Psychologist James Pennebaker has written an influential book called *Opening Up: The Healing Power of Expressing Emotions*. This book documents how talking to people,

HECTOR'S RESPONSIBILITY CHART FOR HIS CHRONIC SKIN RASH

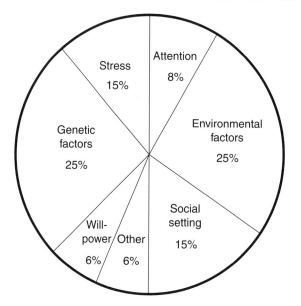

but especially writing, about an upsetting problem can have highly beneficial effects on physical and psychological well-being. In dozens of experiments, Pennebaker and colleagues have shown that spending even 15 minutes a day writing about a currently disturbing situation or experience can have positive emotional effects. Although writing about a difficult experience can cause some temporary increase in negative emotion immediately after a person completes the exercise, within a few hours this disappears. For the majority of individuals, expressive writing leads to positive emotions like relief, happiness, and contentment. It would seem, then, that facing the tigers in your life—that is, actually confronting your feelings about life's failures, losses, and unreasonable demands through expressive writing—can have a positive impact on your emotional state.

Use Repair Strategy 8 when . . .

- you have strong unresolved feelings about a significant loss, failure, or disappointment in your life.
- you have difficulty expressing your feelings.
- you can't talk about a negative situation.

- you try to avoid even thinking about things that bother you.

- you can't stop thinking about a difficult or upsetting problem, situation, or individual.

REPAIR STRATEGY 8 INSTRUCTIONS

According to Pennebaker, there are several steps you need to follow to benefit from expressive writing.

1. **Write on a topic that is a current concern.** It could be a situation that is presently playing itself out in your life, or something that happened in the past that you are still spending a lot of time thinking about.

2. **Write about the objective experience of what happened (i.e., what was said and done by whom and where), but also** *let go* **and write about your very deepest thoughts and feelings about the experience.** What do you feel about the situation and why? What are the effects of the situation on you right now? What are the possible consequences or implications of the situation for you?

3. **You should write continuously, without concern about grammar, spelling, or sentence structure.** Set aside a standard length of time, such as 15 minutes, and stick to that time interval. If you run out of things to write about, repeat what you've already written.

4. **Your writing should be private and not shared with anyone else.** This will ensure that you truly express your deepest thoughts and feelings. Pennebaker also suggests that you do expressive writing for 3–4 consecutive days and then stop for a while. Don't keep a daily diary and write about everything that happens to you. Instead, reserve your expressive writing for situations that are truly upsetting and causing low mood.

Expressive writing counteracts the tendency to avoid or inhibit thinking about a disturbing situation, which is a poor coping strategy associated with more negative mood. It also provides an opportunity to express unwanted intrusive thoughts, which will reduce the impact of these thoughts on your mood state.

TOOL FINDER   See Chapter 1 for an explanation of why thought suppression is counterproductive in mood repair.

People often find new meaning about difficult situations through expressive writing. You might discover a new way to change the situation, minimize its negative impact, or gain new understanding about how to cope.

> **CAUTION** Expressive writing is not the same as journaling. Over the years, I've had many patients who've engaged in daily journaling of their experiences for an extended period of time. Often the practice loses its beneficial effects. Expressive writing should not become a habit. It should be reserved for situations that are truly bothersome and dragging down your mood state. When you do expressive writing, stop after a few days and then don't do it again until you are confronted with another distressing situation. In this way, you will preserve the freshness of expressive writing and avoid turning it into a mundane, routine task.

▶ Repair Strategy ⑨: Take a New Perspective on the Tiger

I have been happily married for close to 40 years, but like all couples, we do have our times when significant differences of opinion arise. Recently we had one of these incidents that became quite heated. In the midst of our argument, I could feel myself becoming intensely upset, defensive, and accusatory, trapped in my own perspective on the problem. I catastrophized about the impact our argument might have on our relationship, but the more I tried to bring it to a close, the further we drifted from any resolution. Finally, after several minutes of silence, I asked myself, "What would I advise an arguing couple in my office? How might I approach the situation with them?" Once I thought about our argument from a different perspective, I was able to gain some new insights into what was happening in our interaction. I changed my way of responding, and we were able to work through the incident.

Sometimes the difficulties in our daily lives are like tigers that seem to pop up out of nowhere. We may be going along as usual when something bad happens; its suddenness throws us off; and we react badly, because we do not truly understand the nature of the difficulty. On the other hand, we can get emotionally attached to the everyday problems that depress us. We become so self-focused, so concerned with the long-term negative consequences, that we easily become blind to possible solutions. We become invested in a certain way of dealing with the problem and can't think cre-

> Taking the long view on a problem or seeing it from the perspective of an outsider can bring new insights and reduce feelings of despair.

atively; we can't think of alternative ways to cope. In other words, we are caught in our own perspective, our own way of understanding the problem. This narrow view can hinder us from changing the situation or finding some other solution. Dealing with either a sudden, unexpected difficulty or a problem that has been around a long time requires that we stand back and try to gain perspective on the problem, trying to see it from another perspective.

Use Repair Strategy 9 when . . .

- you're feeling overwhelmed by either a sudden or a long-standing problem or difficult situation.
- family and friends believe you are overreacting.
- you're preoccupied or worried about the negative consequences of the situation for yourself or your loved ones.
- you're struggling with feelings of uncertainty due to a negative event or situation.

REPAIR STRATEGY 9 INSTRUCTIONS

To help people broaden their insight into a problem, cognitive therapists often use an intervention called *perspective taking*. You can apply this strategy to any tiger that may be lying in wait for you, especially the sudden, unexpected twists and turns of life that leave you with a strong sense of uncertainty about the future.

1. **Imagine that your problem is happening to a friend or family member.** What advice would you give your friend? How might you suggest he/she deal with the problem? How might you understand the problem from the perspective of an outsider, someone who is not struggling with the problematic situation?

2. **Now change the time perspective on the problem.** Ask yourself: "Will this problem be significant in 5 years? What is its likely long-term impact? Am I exaggerating the significant, long-term consequences of this problem?"

    There is a phrase that I often repeat to myself when confronted with a difficult situation: "This too shall pass." It may sound like an oversimplification, but reminding

> Depressive mood increases when you believe that your life is intolerable. Gaining a more realistic perspective can remind you that time heals, that problems are not eternal, and that your resilience is greater than you think.

yourself that everything changes has considerable power to curb your distress over a problem that seems, in the moment, as if it will never end and will only make your life unbearable.

When I was a high school student in the late 1960s, I got into intense arguments with my parents over my long hair and "hippie" clothes. My mother, in particular, was convinced that people would think I was a drug addict and war protester, which was a horrific prospect for her. I was neither. If only she had gained time perspective and realized I was going through an adolescent rebellious phase that would pass quickly with no lasting effects, we could have avoided much emotional turmoil and upset.

Lois was deeply disturbed by her 18-year-old son's drinking. He was not coming home drunk, and there was no evidence of his driving under the influence of alcohol, but she could detect that he had been drinking when he came home late on the weekends. She tried talking to him, but they ended up having verbal arguments that only made her feel more depressed. Her husband thought she was overreacting, so he was no help. One night after church, Lois confided to a friend about her concern with her son's drinking. She discovered that this mother also had a son who drank, but that her friend's feelings about it differed from hers. The two women started to share their experiences, and slowly Lois began to see the problem of underage drinking from a broader perspective. She realized that thousands (if not millions) of parents across North America were facing this problem, and that most teenagers did not become alcoholics or die in horrible car accidents because of alcohol misuse. As she considered how other parents were facing this problem and what the long-term effects for most people were, she began to gain a healthier perspective on the problem. This had a significant impact on her coping strategy and emotional response to her son's behavior. Often we need to readjust our perspective on a problem before we can take action and deal with it effectively.

➤➤➤➤ ➡ Repair Strategy **⑩**: Tame the Tiger by Taking Action

The mood repair strategies presented previously in this chapter should lead to this final outcome, which is taking action—doing something to change a situation or experience that is contributing to your depressed mood. This can be viewed as a "taming of the tiger": You take control of it by refusing to be the victim of the negativity, losses, disappointments, and mistakes that assault you in daily life. For years cognitive behavior therapists have been teaching depressed and anxious patients a set of coping skills, called *problem solving*, for reducing stressors in their lives. Now you can use the same skills as a mood repair strategy to change a situation that is causing you to feel depressed. Often the most effective way to repair sadness is to deal more effectively with the problems and people causing the misery in your life.

Use Repair Strategy 10 when . . .

- there is a person, situation, or circumstance that has a negative effect on your mood state.

- other mood repair strategies will not be helpful unless the life problem is dealt with more effectively.

- your happiness and well-being cannot improve without some resolution of the life problem.

REPAIR STRATEGY 10 INSTRUCTIONS

Problem solving has been described in a number of self-help manuals (see the Resources section of this book), but here I offer a brief overview of a six-step problem-solving approach.

1. *Define the problem:* **Before you can tackle a problematic situation, you need to have a clear understanding of its nature.** Describe the problem in specific, behavioral terms, rather than in terms of vague and generalized feelings. Complex problems need to be broken down into specific parts that you can focus on one at a time. You should use one or two names or phrases for the problem that will help keep you focused on it. For example, doing poorly in school could be defined as "missing classes" and "not studying between classes." The problem of poor physical health could become "not exercising" and "having poor dietary habits." And feeling guilty about your spiritual life could become "not going to church" and "not spending time in prayer and meditation."

2. *Set goals for change:* **Create a very specific, concrete, and realistic description of how you would like the situation to change.** How could the situation change in a way that would make you feel less depressed? How would you like to handle the situation, and what is the most desirable realistic outcome? If the problem that depresses you is "poor physical health," what would be specific indications that you were now in better health?

3. *Brainstorm solutions:* **Write down as many different solutions to the problem as you can think of, without prejudging or evaluating which ones are best.** It's important that you put your censor on hold; be open-minded and creative, writing down any solution you can think of, no matter how ridiculous it may seem.

For example, Rachel, who was normally athletic, was feeling depressed by her poor physical fitness after recovering from surgery. She identified her problem as "reduced physical fitness" and "limited ability to exercise." Her goal was to regain her presurgery fitness level and return to running 10K races. Her brainstorming solutions included the following: start running long distances as soon as possible, abandon any attempt to run again, take out membership in a gym, hire a personal trainer, build up her physical stamina gradually, settle on running short distances, or switch to biking.

4. *Evaluate each solution:* **Examine the solutions you have brainstormed, and write down the pros/cons or the advantages/disadvantages of each.** Rachel realized that trying to run long distances immediately, giving up her passion for running, and switching to biking were all unrealistic. Each of the other solutions had advantages and disadvantages, so she selected the one for her action plan that seemed to have the most advantages and the fewest disadvantages (i.e., hire a personal trainer and work on a physical strengthening program).

5. *Implement an action plan:* **After selecting a solution, break it down into various components or tasks that you will need to implement in order to try it out.** Describe what you need to do, when you will do it, and any problems you might encounter doing the task. Then record whether or not you tried it. Rachel's action plan for starting a physical strengthening program included asking friends for recommendations, checking out various gyms, searching online for postsurgery recovery programs, consulting with her surgeon about physical exercise, meeting with a physical trainer, completing a prefitness assessment, and scheduling her first week of fitness training.

6. *Evaluate the outcome:* **Problem solving does not end with taking action.** It is important to proceed to this final step and actually determine whether your course of action has been effective, or at least whether you are on the right track. There are two outcomes that are important to consider. First, has the solution you chose led to the type of change in the problem you desire? And second, how has the process of implementing the solution—the action plan—affected your mood? Do you feel more or less depressed by the action you've taken? You may decide that you've selected the right action plan, but now need to persist longer to meet your goals. Or you may decide that the solution was not the right one, and so you need to go back, select another solution, and develop a different course of action. After 1 week on her strengthening program, Rachel felt a lot of aches and pain, and was still a long way from her presurgery fitness level. However, she knew that it was too early to evaluate the effectiveness of her action plan, and so she decided

to give it until the end of the month. She did note that she felt less depressed, because at least now she was doing something about her poor physical fitness.

Depressed Mood, Negative Situations, and So Much More

There can be little doubt that what happens to us in our daily lives has a profound impact on our moods. All of us have tigers in our lives—experiences that come our way unexpectedly (maybe even tragically), or long-term situations that seem to have no possibility of resolution. Either way, they leave us feeling vulnerable, victimized by circumstances, depressed, and discouraged. If you find yourself in a funk or feeling blue, it is likely that some negative event involving a sense of loss, failure, disappointment, or helplessness is dragging down your mood state. Dealing with these "tigers" is an important aspect of repairing depressed mood. This chapter has presented a variety of coping strategies you can use to modify the effects of negative situations and rescue yourself from the blues.

Whether our experiences involve sudden or long-term major life events, or the annoying, trivial things that happen on a daily basis, personal circumstances and situations do not affect our moods directly. Rather, the way we think about and evaluate the events and situations in our lives determines whether we feel happy or sad. This evaluation is called *appraisal*, and it is well known to emotion researchers that how we appraise experiences determines how we feel. Depressed mood is associated with situations that we evaluate as involving some loss, failure, or uncontrollable occurrence. Changing the way we think about negative situations, ourselves, and our ability to cope is a powerful approach to repairing depressed mood. The next chapter presents a set of mood repair strategies that psychologists have found highly effective in treating people with severe forms of clinical depression. You will want to use the cognitive strategies in the next chapter together with the situation change interventions in this chapter to strengthen your efforts at depressive mood repair.

4 silence the inner critic

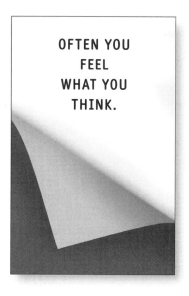

OFTEN YOU FEEL WHAT YOU THINK.

Although she was a highly successful human resources consultant with a promising career, Christine suffered from recurring bouts of negative mood that often lasted several days. Despite being tearful and feeling lethargic, she always made it to work. But if it wasn't enough that she found it hard to concentrate and get things done at her usual rate, she also beat herself up for feeling down and not being able to pull herself out of her funk. During these times of intense sadness, Christine's thinking became much darker, more negative, and cynical. She withdrew from family and friends, and she spent a lot of time in bed ruminating about the things that were missing from her life, particularly a life partner. She would review past relationships and go over and over the reasons she might have been rejected: She was "fat and ugly," or "too cold and awkward around men." Her self-blame and self-loathing inevitably led her to conclude that her life was pointless and that her future would be lonely and miserable. Christine's entire outlook on the world, herself, her life circumstances, and her future turned exceedingly negative. During her low moods, it was as if Christine were on trial within her own mind, and a particularly harsh judge had weighed the evidence and determined that her life was a complete failure. For Christine, learning to silence her inner critic was an important part of mood repair.

Are You Overwhelmed by Negativity?

Our ability to live and function in this world depends on the brain's capacity to process information every moment of the day. This means that we constantly think about what is happening around us, about other people and ourselves, and about how we should behave and respond to all the demands of life. One unique characteristic of being

human is our ability to be self-conscious—to think about and evaluate ourselves, to consider how we might appear to others, and to ponder the outcomes of our actions. Our self-consciousness also means that we are aware of our thoughts and so have considerable ability to direct or control our thinking processes toward achieving important tasks. To write these sentences about the human mind, for example, I need to exert some control over my thought processes. I need to concentrate on thinking about the subject at hand—human cognition—and not allow myself to get distracted by thinking about the weather, what I will be doing 2 hours from now, or some upsetting event that happened last week. I also need to control any distracting thoughts that might involve self-evaluation, such as "This is probably no good," "What if my editors think this is drivel?", and "This is not making any sense." In other words, *silencing the inner critic* is essential to achieving my writing objective.

> Thinking about loss and failure will make you feel sad, whereas thinking about success and acceptance will make you feel happy.

This inner critic is fueled by automatic negative thoughts that mutter beneath the surface of our consciousness, making it hard to heed well-intentioned advice to "look on the bright side" and "think more positively." As explained in the sidebar "The Discovery of Depressive Thinking" on pages 52–53, negative thoughts are highly credible simply because they are consistent with our negative feelings when stuck in the blues. So even if you force yourself to think positively, it seems ridiculous or unbelievable, and thus the positive thoughts don't stick; they don't change the way you feel. This is why learning to silence the inner critic becomes important work: It must be undertaken so that more positive, realistic thinking can emerge and repair depressed mood. The following are some examples of the negative thinking that we find so credible but that only makes us feel worse. Do any of these look familiar to you? Although these examples may look extreme to you, are these familiar themes voiced by your inner critic?

"Everything I try to do ends in failure and disappointment."

"I have no talents or abilities."

"I'm such a failure in life."

"My life will never improve; I'm stuck with a miserable existence."

"No one really cares about what happens to me."

"People don't like me; they don't want to be around me."

the discovery of depressive thinking

In the early 1960s, Aaron T. Beck, a professor of psychiatry at the University of Pennsylvania Medical School, made an important discovery while using psychoanalysis to treat his depressed patients. Beck had asked his patients to report any thoughts that entered their mind during the therapy session. He discovered that his patients actually had two streams of thought, which occurred simultaneously. The first stream consisted of thoughts that people were highly aware of and that dealt with the task at hand, such as "I need to tell Dr. Beck about my bad week," or "I think I should talk about my demanding mother." Psychiatrists focused their interpretive skills on these highly conscious thoughts. But Beck discovered a second stream of thinking that was unintended, more automatic, and just barely noticeable to his patients. He labeled this type of thinking *automatic thoughts*. With some effort and training, Beck was able to teach his patients to refocus their attention on these automatic thoughts.

What he discovered was that people with clinical depression were frequently having very negative automatic thoughts about themselves, their personal circumstances, and their future—thoughts that they hardly knew existed. So in the therapy sessions, as they were talking about their distressing weeks or difficult childhoods, they were also having automatic thoughts like "I don't think I am doing this right," "I'm probably the most hopeless case Dr. Beck has seen," and "He probably thinks I'm such a complainer." What Beck discovered in his depressed patients was a highly critical inner voice that was barely noticeable because it occurred at the level of a whisper, yet had a profound impact on directing the course of their depression.

Over the next two decades Beck worked on developing a form of talk therapy, called *cognitive therapy*, which has proven highly effective in correcting exaggerated negative automatic thoughts and relieving the symptoms of clinical depression. The key elements of this therapy form the core of the strategies in this chapter, which will help you learn to silence your inner critic and repair your depressed mood.

Beck's groundbreaking discoveries shifted the research direction of psychologists and psychiatrists toward understanding more about how people think when they are feeling depressed. This is what we've learned after 50 years of this clinical research:

- *We all have automatic thoughts*, although we may have to be trained to become aware of this type of thinking.
- *The way we think affects the way we feel*. Whether our depressed mood is brief and mild or long-lasting and severe, our automatic thoughts are overwhelmingly negative, whereas we tend to have positive automatic thoughts when we are feeling happy or joyful.

- *Negative automatic thoughts are almost always exaggerated, biased reflections of reality.* When we are feeling sad or depressed, our negative automatic thoughts become preoccupied with loss and failure, so we become highly self-critical. Because of their one-sided focus, the automatic thoughts during depressed mood are poor and inaccurate reflections of our self-worth and personal circumstances.

- *There are three types of automatic thoughts during depressed mood:* a *negative self-view,* in which we dwell on our inadequacies, defects, and worthlessness; a *negative world view,* in which our personal circumstances are seen in terms of defeat or deprivation; and a *negative view of the future,* in which we expect future difficulty, suffering, and deprivation.

- *Negative thinking is highly self-focused and evaluative in nature.* We evaluate our worth, often by comparing ourselves unfavorably to others along measures of good versus bad, loved versus unloved, successful versus failing, and the like. The thoughts may focus on situations in our lives that confirm our sense of ourselves as unloved, rejected, or incompetent. We end up stuck on our most negative attributes.

- *Negative automatic thinking dominates because it is so believable.* Because it matches our negative mood states, we find our negative thinking believable, making it more difficult to accept a positive outlook.

"There's nothing I can do; I'm too weak and ineffective."

"I can't trust or depend on anyone."

Cognitive Mood Repair

Changing the way you think requires a systematic approach that was first developed by Aaron T. Beck for the treatment of clinical depression (again, see the sidebar above). Known as *cognitive restructuring,* the intervention involves several steps that I have divided into four strategies. You will need to do Repair Strategies 11, 12, and 13 in the sequence recommended, ending with Repair Strategy 14. Although your work on Repair Strategies 11–13 might lead to some improved mood, you should always end with Repair Strategy 14, which is accepting a more balanced, alternative way of thinking.

Use cognitive mood repair when . . .

- your mind is filled with negative thinking about yourself, your future, or your personal circumstances.
- it is difficult to think about your life in a more balanced, rational manner.
- you believe the inner critic.
- you can't simply distract yourself from negative thinking, but instead get stuck in it.

⟫⟫⟫ Repair Strategy ⓫: Know the Critic

The first step in silencing the inner critic is to know how you are criticizing yourself. Certain negative critical thoughts tend to recur during periods of sadness. Fortunately, you can train yourself to be more aware of the inner critical voice, so you can deal with one of the key sources of your negative mood state.

REPAIR STRATEGY 11 INSTRUCTIONS

1. **Start by tracking your negative mood states. Take a blank sheet of paper and create a Negative Thought Record like the partial form shown on the facing page, or print out a complete form from *www.guilford.com/clark7-forms*.**
   The main purpose of this tracking form is to capture the negative thoughts that occur during your low mood states. So most of your work will focus on the last column.

2. **After creating your Negative Thought Record, begin by writing down any circumstances, events, or situations that happened to you during the day that might have triggered your depressed mood.** In the first column, you should also record the date and time each situation occurred. One of the best ways to capture negative thinking is to focus on thoughts associated with a problematic event, person, or situation.

3. **Next, rate the intensity of your sadness associated with the situation on a 10-point scale, where 0 = no sadness and 10 = the deepest sadness you have ever felt.**

4. **Finally, start work on the last column by asking yourself certain questions about your emotional state, such as "Why am I feeling down right now?", "Has anything happened today that disappoints me?", and "Have I been criticized,**

Negative Thought Record

Date and time	Situation related to depressed mood	Intensity of depressed mood (0–10)	Negative thoughts (my inner critical voice)

let down, or discouraged in any way?" Then ask yourself, "What is bothering me about this situation or circumstance?", "How is this affecting me negatively?", and "What is so discouraging or upsetting about this situation?". It is important to jot down your answers to these questions in the "Negative Thoughts" column, and then to ask yourself:

"What am I thinking about myself right now in regard to this situation?"

"Am I blaming myself—holding myself responsible for this negative event or circumstance?"

"Am I thinking about the negative consequences, or maybe even catastrophizing the future?"

"Am I thinking that this will have an enduring negative effect on all aspects of my life?"

The point of these questions is to "drill down" to the deeper automatic thoughts that reflect what you believe about yourself, your worth, and your value as a human being. The ultimate questions deal with your critical evaluation of your self-worth:

"What am I thinking is so bad about me?"

"What disappoints me about myself?"

"What do I dislike most about myself?"

"What would I desperately like to change in myself?"

> What are your self-critical issues—
> the negative things about yourself
> that you automatically think
> when you are feeling depressed?
> Identifying this type of thinking is
> key to overcoming low mood.

These deeper critical automatic thoughts about the self are often triggered by negative events and are responsible for maintaining a state of depressed mood and discouragement.

Most people who struggle with depressed mood have one or more recurring critical themes that get triggered when discouragement comes their way. Often the inner critic focuses on issues such as incompetence, failure, rejection, disapproval, not being loved, abandonment, shame, embarrassment, and loss. Negative situations at work, school, relationships, health, finances, and even leisure or recreation can elicit these critical automatic thoughts about yourself. The first step toward overcoming the inner critical voice and repairing your depressed mood is to know how you are being harsh on yourself. What is your self-critical theme? What do you dislike most about yourself?

Christine noticed that she often felt most depressed when she stayed at work late and then came home to an empty apartment, hungry and too tired to cook a decent meal. In the "Situation . . . " column of the Negative Thought Record, she wrote, "Sitting alone in my apartment, eating leftover Chinese takeout, and watching a stupid reality program about love and romance." She rated her depressed mood as 7 of a possible 10. In the "Negative Thoughts" column, she wrote, "I am sitting here all alone," "Other people have someone in their life, but not me," "All I have is my work and nothing more," "My life is so empty and pathetic outside of work," "I am living a useless existence," "I am so lonely and miserable," and "I'll probably end up alone and miserable the rest of my life, and it's all my fault for being so fat and lazy." Notice that Christine started by writing down thoughts about her situation (coming home to an empty apartment), but as she drilled down to what she was thinking about herself, the really depressing thoughts were about being alone and miserable for the rest of her life and blaming herself for her life circumstances. It was these deeper automatic thoughts, which cognitive therapists call "hot thoughts," that Christine had to correct to repair her depressed mood. What are the hot critical thoughts that dominate your mind during periods of sadness or dysphoria? Learning to become more aware of the inner critical voice during periods of dysphoria is an important step in negative mood repair. You may begin to question the negative thoughts once you see on paper just how negative and one-sided they are. This can result in some mood improvement, but you should continue with the rest of the exercises in this chapter for more stable mood change.

➤➤➤ Repair Strategy ⑫: Weigh the Facts

Once you have discovered the recurring negative theme in the thoughts voiced by your inner critic, the next step is to evaluate its accuracy. How does your thinking compare with real life? *What is the evidence for and against your negative critical self-evaluation?* Although there may be lots of evidence of imperfection in your life, are you exaggerating your negative qualities or the seriousness of the situation? Learning to challenge your negative automatic thoughts—to correct them so that they more accurately reflect reality—is the most potent cognitive therapy intervention for repairing depressed mood. We call this therapy technique *evidence gathering,* and you can use the form below to do this type of mood repair work.

> Realistic thinking is a great antidote for depressed mood. Evidence gathering is the best way to determine how far your thinking is from the standard of reality.

REPAIR STRATEGY 12 INSTRUCTIONS

1. In the space provided at the top of the Evidence-Gathering Form (a partial form is shown below, or you can print out a complete one from *www.guilford.*

Evidence–Gathering Form

Record your self-critical "hot thought": _____

_____

Evidence that confirms the self-critical thought	Evidence that refutes the self-critical thought
1.	1.
2.	2.

com/clark7-forms), **write down the main self-critical thought that you discovered from doing the preceding exercise (Repair Strategy 11).** This should be the thought that most often occurs during your periods of negative mood and is most distressing to you. Make sure it is a self-criticism that you are still experiencing and that continues to cause you much distress.

2. **Now ask yourself what has occurred that would make you believe this self-critical thought to be accurate. Write down your answers in the left-hand column on the form ("Evidence That Confirms . . . ").**

3. **Then ask yourself what evidence refutes this thought—what would be a more realistic way to view this subject—and write it in the right-hand column of the form ("Evidence That Refutes . . . ").**

As an example, let's examine Julie's core self-critical thought about her physical appearance, which caused her to feel depressed and discouraged because she couldn't seem to lose weight. When feeling depressed, Julie was highly self-critical, thinking of herself in derogatory terms—for instance, "I'm disgustingly fat and ugly because I'm too lazy to diet and exercise." The first things that Julie needed to ask herself were these: "What has happened to me that makes me think I'm fat and ugly because I'm lazy?" and "In what way is my thinking about physical beauty and weight loss accurate?" She wrote down answers to these questions in the first column in support of the self-critical thought. Then she proceeded to the second column and wrote down evidence against the critical thought by asking herself, "Does anything from my experience suggest that the self-critical thought is inaccurate or exaggerated?" and "What is a more realistic, accurate way to think about physical beauty and weight loss?" The filled-out example for Julie shown on pages 59–60 illustrates some possible evidence-gathering responses to Julie's negative automatic thought.

The main point of this mood repair strategy is to gather evidence that the negative self-critical automatic thought is an exaggeration that does not match reality. Obviously, there is always some grain of truth to a self-criticism. A little self-criticism is not the problem and can actually be beneficial. What maintains depressed mood is self-criticism that becomes excessive, inaccurate, and biased. And so the way to repair depressed mood is to correct the exaggerated self-criticism so that it becomes more realistic. Evidence gathering is not a quick fix. It will take practice to use this strategy to repair depressed mood. But give it a try. See whether you feel a little better, a little less depressed, when you correct the inner critic with evidence from real life.

Evidence-Gathering Form: Julie

Evidence that confirms the self-critical thought	Evidence that refutes the self-critical thought
1. I've tried repeated diets, but failed to maintain weight loss.	1. I have successfully lost weight with many of my diets, but couldn't maintain the weight loss.
2. I've joined the gym so many times, and then I never go more than a few times.	2. I've never been athletic, so why should I think that I would start when I'm 45 years old?
3. I am 50 pounds overweight.	3. I actually weighed more a few years right after my kids were born, so I have done a little better in keeping the weight down.
4. I end up eating food that I know I should not be eating.	4. It is true that I often eat the wrong food, but I have reduced the amount of fast food I eat, and I rarely have dessert.
5. I rarely get compliments about my physical appearance.	5. How often does the average woman get compliments about her physical appearance? Maybe I'm being unrealistic in how often people get compliments. Also, maybe I get occasional compliments but don't notice them.
6. My husband has lost interest in me sexually.	6. How much is the lack of sexual interest due to my physical appearance, and how much to our increasing age and busy, stressful lifestyle?
	7. Compared to the average middle-aged woman, how unattractive and overweight am I? I know I'm a long way from a beauty queen, but is my physical appearance closer to the average than I think?
	8. Am I exaggerating the importance of beauty and weight loss for my happiness? My job and family are more important to my life satisfaction than my physical appearance.
	9. I've actually been quite disciplined when I diet. Like everyone who has dieted, the big challenge is maintaining the weight loss.

Evidence that confirms the self-critical thought	Evidence that refutes the self-critical thought
	10. I'm really not a lazy or undisciplined person. I've been successful in my job and have successfully juggled work and family life.
	11. I do get compliments from my close female friends when I wear a new outfit.

➤➤➤ Repair Strategy ⓭: Know Your Biases

How we see ourselves, our life circumstances, the future, or even other people is never completely accurate. Our past influences how we see the present and imagine the future. Some people are by nature more positive and optimistic, tending to focus on their positive characteristics and expecting that things will turn out fine. Other people are by nature more negative and pessimistic, focusing on their negative characteristics and thinking about the possibility of bad future outcomes. Whichever group you fall into, the way you see yourself and the world can't be perfectly clear and accurate. We all see things through somewhat clouded lenses, and we naturally tend toward seeing either the rosy or the darkly tinted side of things. And as we process information and try to understand ourselves, the world around us, and our relationships, we all make *cognitive errors*, or mistakes in our thinking. These cognitive errors are especially evident when we are feeling down or depressed.

Beck and his colleagues have identified several cognitive errors that people tend to make when they are feeling down. These errors contribute to our tendency to make negative evaluations and raise the volume on the voice of the inner critic.

- *All-or-nothing thinking:* the tendency to view yourself, others, and even situations in black-or-white categories with no grays (e.g., thinking of yourself as highly competent only if you succeed in absolutely everything you do, or as a complete failure if you struggle in even one area of your life).

- *Negative filtering:* the tendency to see only the negative aspects of people or situations, and to ignore the positive elements (e.g., dwelling on a critical remark by a coworker, while not even being able to remember the friendly and complimentary comments of others).

- *Personalization:* the tendency to assume that you are responsible for negative events or other people's bad behavior, and therefore to excessively blame your-self rather than others or external circumstances (e.g., your friend Marla makes a curt remark, and you assume that you must have angered her rather than that she might be having a bad day).

- *Overgeneralization*: the tendency to jump to conclusions—that is, to make a broad generalization from a single incident or situation (e.g., assuming your marriage is in trouble after a heated verbal disagreement over finances).

- *Catastrophizing*: the tendency to anticipate the worst in the future, without considering less negative possible outcomes (e.g., being convinced that you'll lose your job and will have to foreclose on your mortgage when your company has announced that it is restructuring).

- *Imperatives (i.e., shoulds)*: the tendency to judge yourself or others in terms of rigid, fixed ideas or expectations (e.g., expecting people always to treat you in a polite and fair manner).

REPAIR STRATEGY 13 INSTRUCTIONS

Becoming aware of your cognitive errors, and then trying to come up with a more bal-anced way of thinking, constitute a powerful strategy for repairing depressed mood.

1. **Using the Negative Thought Record you filled out earlier, see whether you can identify any cognitive errors in your negative thinking when you are feeling down or discouraged.**

2. **Then, whenever you do feel down or depressed, ask yourself these questions:**

    "What thinking errors am I making as I reflect on this situation or as I think about myself?"

    "Are these errors leading me to draw overly negative, critical conclusions about myself or life circumstances?"

    "What would be a more accurate way to think about these events?"

Cognitive therapists have found that learning to catch and correct cognitive errors can lead to improvements in negative mood states.

George had recently retired from a successful law firm and moved with his wife to a new home in southern Florida. George had struggled most of his life with depressed mood and irritability, but this intensified after his retirement. Despite the promise of the "golden years," George's deteriorating mood state was causing extreme hardship for the couple. As George started to track his negative and irritable mood episodes, he discovered that a common self-critical theme in his thinking was "I have no purpose, no use any more—I am losing my abilities and becoming a useless old man." George soon began to identify several errors in his depressive thinking. He was seeing himself and his retirement in *all-or-nothing terms*; that is, he felt that once he was no longer practicing law, he was useless, of no value. He was also overly focused on the negative (*negative filtering*); that is, he believed that he was doing nothing useful or productive during the day. In addition, he held several *imperatives* or *shoulds*: "Your worth or value should depend on productive work," "If you don't work, you shouldn't expect anything," and "People should agree with your point of view." Finally, George was *catastrophizing*, seeing his senior years as simply a waiting period for death.

►►► Repair Strategy 14: Discover an Alternative Way of Thinking

If you have practiced the first three mood repair strategies in this chapter, you are ready to learn how to develop a more balanced, realistic way of thinking about yourself, your life circumstances, and other people. In fact, your work on the previous exercises may already have led you to consider a more realistic way of thinking than the negative automatic thoughts that trigger low mood. Becoming skilled at correcting the overly negative inner critic and replacing it with a more reasonable, balanced perspective is an especially powerful tool for repairing negative or depressed mood. This essential element of cognitive therapy is one of the factors that has made it such an effective treatment for clinical depression.

REPAIR STRATEGY 14 INSTRUCTIONS

1. **Review the Evidence-Gathering Form that you completed earlier. Carefully consider the evidence for and against the self-critical "hot thought."**

2. **As you look at the evidence for and against your negative thinking, how exaggerated is the hot thought? What is a more realistic alternative way of thinking about yourself or the situation?**

3. **Write down the alternative way of thinking at the bottom of the form.** In fact, you may come up with two or three alternative ways of thinking. However, make sure that the alternatives are specific to the thought recorded on the form, that they recognize both positive and negative aspects of the situation, and that they are more realistic than the negative "hot thought."

4. **Adopt a "therapist's perspective" when constructing your alternative. That is,**

strive for a viewpoint that recognizes both the positive and negative things about yourself, your circumstances, or your problems. Ask yourself how a friend or mental health therapist might view the situation. Try to see yourself or the situation from a third-party perspective: What would this other person advise you in terms of how to think about the situation?

To illustrate generating an alternative, let's take Julie's negative thought, "I'm disgustingly fat and ugly because I'm too lazy to diet and exercise." Of course we can see several cognitive errors in this type of thinking, such as all-or-nothing thinking, catastrophizing, negative filtering, and even overgeneralization. As we look at the evidence-gathering exercise, we can see several more balanced and realistic ways that Julie could think about her physical appearance. Of course, she couldn't deny that she was overweight, because she knew that this was true. However, Julie might think back to times when she weighed more and realize that she was not actually as overweight now as she had been in the past. In other words, she had made some progress on losing weight, although she was still not yet at her desired weight level. Also, she could remind herself that she had succeeded in maintaining some weight loss over a long period of time, and that anyone who has dieted knows that keeping the weight off is a lot harder than losing pounds.

Another thing that Julie might realize through evidence gathering was that she was placing too much importance on physical beauty. She realized that all she really wanted was to look nice, more like the average middle-aged American woman. This would be a long way from her exaggerated self-criticism that she was "disgustingly fat and ugly" and "too lazy." So Julie came up with a more realistic, balanced perspective:

> "It is true that I am overweight and have struggled with dieting for many years. However, I have had some success with weight loss, so clearly I am not lazy or lacking in discipline. I also don't need beauty to be confident and satisfied with myself. All I need to accept my appearance is to believe I look as nice as most middle-aged women. So my goal needs to be to improve my physical health through some changes I could make in my diet and daily exercise, and to work on celebrating the small successes I make in this part of my life."

Once Julie developed this balanced, realistic way of thinking about her weight and physical appearance, she felt less depressed and discouraged. Evidence gathering and developing alternatives became key mood repair strategies that Julie used to lift herself out of despair over her physical appearance.

It will take time and practice for you to become skilled at generating alternatives. At first you may find the alternatives dubious or hard to believe, because they challenge your old, critical way of thinking. Try to remember that these doubts are coming

the mood induction experiment

In recent years, psychologists have conducted numerous experiments to discover the most effective ways to reduce sadness. My colleagues and I have conducted some of this research in our own lab, and there is agreement that a mood regulation strategy called *cognitive reappraisal* can significantly reduce the intensity of sadness within minutes. Cognitive reappraisal involves changing the meaning of a situation, or how people think about its consequences or their ability to cope with it, so as to change its emotional impact. In the lab experiments, participants were shown a short film clip that caused them to feel sad (such as a film involving a tragic death), and were asked either to imagine that this had happened to a loved one or to view the film as fictitious. Those who imagined this happening to a loved one were quite sad, while those who viewed the film as fiction experienced reduced sadness. In your own life, you can do the same thing by recasting the meaning of a situation or problem.

Julie, for example, reappraised her weight as a problem that she could manage better than she thought. She decided that she could allow herself some increased weight and still maintain confidence and self-worth, and that she could live a satisfied life as a physically average middle-aged woman. This reappraisal reduced the influence of the inner critic on Julie's emotional state. Her mood improved, because now she was able to think more realistically about a few changes she could make in her diet and physical exercise. The inner critic was silenced, so her weight loss goals became more realistic and she began learning to accept herself at a larger size, since she was coming to believe that physical beauty really wasn't the most important thing in her life.

from your inner critic, and keep practicing. As you practice countering your negative thoughts with more realistic, balanced thinking, you will become more comfortable with the process, allowing you to experience substantial mood repair effects. The ability to change feelings by changing the way you think has been demonstrated scientifically, as discussed above in the sidebar "The Mood Induction Experiment."

➤➤➤ Repair Strategy **⑮**: Consider the Consequences

As you work on correcting your negative thinking, there is a very practical view you can take of cognitive mood repair. Ask yourself:

"Even if there is some truth to my negative thinking, what effect is this negative perspective having on me, my circumstances, my relationships, and the like?"

"What is it costing me to continue to see myself and life through darkly tinted glasses?"

Use Repair Strategy 15 when . . .

- you're stuck in your negative thinking, despite doing the cognitive mood repair strategies you have learned to this point.

- you want to strengthen your belief in a more realistic alternative way of thinking.

- you're not convinced of the adverse effects of negative thinking on your depression.

It is important that you also recognize the consequences—the cost to you—of continuing to listen to the harsh, critical inner voice versus the new, more adaptive alternative. For example, if your negative thought is "I will never succeed in life," and you've experienced significant failures at work or in your relationships, evidence gathering may still lead you to the negative conclusion. But you can also look at this from a practical perspective: What effect is thinking that you'll never succeed in life having on you right now? Could it cause you to give up, and so you end up fulfilling what you've come to expect? There is a serious cost to assuming "I'll never succeed in life." Would it not be more useful to adopt a more hopeful way of thinking, even if it might not be totally accurate? Cognitive therapists call this *cost/benefit analysis*, and here's how to do it.

REPAIR STRATEGY 15 INSTRUCTIONS

1. **Take a sheet of paper and create the Cost/Benefit Analysis Form shown in part on page 66, or print out a complete one from *www.guilford.com/clark7-forms*.**

2. **Write down the negative automatic or self-critical thought that you intend to evaluate. Now think back to past experiences with this thought.** What have been the positive and negative consequences to you of thinking so critically? What are the short-term and longer-term consequences of having this thought? As you think about the future, what are the consequences of continuing to listen to the harsh inner critic?

3. **Now record the more balanced alternative way of thinking that you intend to evaluate.** Naturally you will not have as much experience with this perspective,

Cost/Benefit Analysis Form

Part A. Record the negative thought you are evaluating: _____

_____

Benefits of accepting the negative thought	Costs of accepting the negative thought
1.	1.
2.	2.

Part B. Record the alternative thought you are evaluating: _____

_____

Benefits of accepting the negative thought	Costs of accepting the negative thought
1.	1.
2.	2.

so you'll have to base your cost/benefit analysis on what you imagine would be the effects of more realistic thinking. List the advantages and disadvantages of thinking more realistically about yourself. What might be the immediate and longer-term consequences of accepting the alternative perspective? In what ways could the future be made better or worse by accepting the alternative way of thinking?

4. **Formulate a conclusion. Based on your Cost/Benefit Analysis Form, is it better to accept the negative or the alternative thinking?** From a purely practical point

of view, is the alternative or your negative thinking the best guide to living? If your conclusion is the alternative thinking provides the most benefit and least cost to you, then repeatedly remind yourself of this conclusion each time you slip into negative thinking and feel depressed.

Doing a cost/benefit analysis of your negative versus your more constructive way of thinking about yourself emphasizes the importance of silencing the critic and listening to the more adaptive, rational perspective on your self-worth, life circumstances, and future. You will find this mood repair strategy most helpful if you keep the Cost/Benefit Analysis Form handy and frequently add to your lists of advantages and disadvantages over several days, or even weeks, as you have different experiences that relate to the negative and alternative thinking.

> **Consider the personal cost of continuing to listen to the critic versus the missed benefits of adopting the healthier alternative.**

Christine did a cost/benefit analysis on her negative automatic thought "I'll be alone and miserable the rest of my life," versus the healthier alternative "I can't predict the future. Many people find love at a variety of ages, and others who remain single are not hopelessly miserable every moment of their lives. I can learn to be more content with my single status." Christine could not think of any advantages to the negative thought, but lots of disadvantages: (1) It caused her to feel depressed and miserable; (2) she isolated herself in her apartment because of it; (3) she constantly complained to family and close friends about her misery; (4) the thought ate away at her self-confidence; (5) it caused her to feel inferior in social situations, so she became too reserved and passive; (6) she avoided social engagements that involved both men and women, thereby limiting her opportunities of meeting a potential date; and (7) she acted cold and aloof around men, giving the unintended message that she was not interested in dating. When it came to the healthier alternative, the only costs that Christine could list were these: (1) "This way of thinking does not feel right or natural," (2) "Maybe I'm trying to believe a falsehood, and I will remain single the rest of my life," and (3) "It takes considerable time and effort to change the way you think and feel." However, she discovered many benefits to adopting the alternative view of herself and her future, such as (1) feeling less depressed about her life circumstances, (2) feeling more confident and outgoing around men, (3) engaging in less self-pity and complaining to others, (4) being more receptive to potential dating opportunities and overtures of interest from men, (5) agreeing to explore adult singles organizations that engaged in interesting activities, (6) considering signing up for an online dating service, and (7) feeling more satisfied and contented with her life.

➤➤➤➤ Repair Strategy 🔟: Take Action against the Critic

You have no doubt heard the phrase "Actions speak louder than words." Nothing could be truer when it comes to mood repair. To truly change the way you think so that you will feel less depressed, you need to change your behavior; that is, you need to act on your new alternative way of thinking. This is the most powerful approach that cognitive therapists use with their depressed patients to shift from negative automatic thinking to more positive, adaptive thinking. We call this *empirical hypothesis testing*, and it is designed to weaken belief in the negative, self-critical thoughts and strengthen belief in the more positive alternative cognitions. Essentially, this involves planning a series of activities that will constitute a test of your negative thinking versus the more realistic alternative. You can use the Action Plan Form shown in part below (or print one out from *www.guilford.com/clark7-forms*) to plan and record your cognitive mood repair activities. You'll also find a table after the Repair Strategy 16 instructions (pp. 70–71), which contains some examples of behavioral action plans that can be used to challenge typical negative thinking.

Action Plan Form

Negative thought evaluated: _____

_____

Alternative thought evaluated: _____

_____

Your action plan	How you carried out the action plan	Action plan outcome

Use Repair Strategy 16 when . . .

- you engage in cognitive mood repair.

- you want to strengthen your acceptance of alternative thoughts.

- you want to reduce your belief in negative, self-critical thinking.

REPAIR STRATEGY 16 INSTRUCTIONS

1. **Select a specific negative thought and write down the consequences of accepting that thought.** For example, let's assume your negative thought is "I can't make decisions, because I always get it wrong." One implication of believing this thought is that you avoid making decisions even on everyday activities like choosing a restaurant. You always leave it up to others to decide where to eat.

2. **Next, think of a routine activity that would directly challenge the negative thought and its implication.** In our example, you could decide to invite friends or family to eat at your favorite Asian restaurant. This activity would be a direct test of your negative belief that you always make poor decisions.

3. **Write out in the first column of the Action Plan Form ("Your Action Plan") specific instructions for how, when, where, and with whom you will implement your activity.** Don't leave anything to chance; be very clear and specific about what you have to do to test the negative thought targeted by your action plan.

4. **Before engaging in the activity, record a positive and a negative outcome expectation.** What would have to happen that would confirm the negative thought, and what outcome of the activity would support the alternative cognition? In our example, your friends' complaining about the restaurant would confirm that you can't make good decisions, whereas evidence that they enjoyed the evening with you at the restaurant would support the alternative thought that sometimes you can make a fine decision.

5. **Engage in the activity, and describe your experience in the second column of the Action Plan Form.** Make sure you record everything you experienced, both positive and negative, as well as aspects of the activity you expected and the things you didn't expect.

6. **Evaluate the outcome of your experience, and record it in the third column of the Action Plan Form.** What was the consequence or outcome of the activity? In our example, how many people accepted your invitation for dinner at the restau-

rant? How was the food? What's the evidence that people did or did not enjoy the evening? Were there any complaints? What is your conclusion—did you make a good decision or not? Is this activity evidence that at least sometimes you can make a good, or at least acceptable, decision?

7. **Using what you've learned from this exercise, how could you change your behavior in a way that challenges the negative thought and reinforces the alternative?** For example, could you plan on making at least three specific decisions a week at work, such as scheduling team meetings, offering your opinion on a project, and inviting colleagues to join you for lunch?

Negative automatic thought	*Behavioral action plan*
"I don't get any pleasure or enjoyment out of life."	Engage in some activities you used to enjoy, and then rate on a 10-point scale how much enjoyment you experienced. You may not have enjoyed the activity as much as you did in the past, but was it true that you felt absolutely no enjoyment (not even a 1/10)?
"I have no friends, because people don't like me due to my frequent negative moods."	Take the initiative and call an acquaintance or a former friend. Invite this person for coffee, a movie, dinner out, or the like, and note the response. Suggest several possible dates so that this person can pick the most convenient time. Make note of the experience and any indication that the person enjoyed the social activity.
"I'm such a failure; I never succeed at anything I try to do."	Initiate a new activity, hobby, or work assignment. Record your experience of learning this new activity and the degree of success you experienced in mastering the activity. Is it true that you utterly fail at everything you try?

Negative automatic thought	*Behavioral action plan*
"I am so unattractive, even ugly; how can I possibly feel satisfied with myself?"	Take note of all the people in your life, and rate each of them on a 10-point scale for physical attractiveness and life satisfaction. Is it true that only the physically attractive are happy in this life? Now take note of strangers, especially couples, you see in stores or on the streets. Is it true that all the physically attractive people look happy and the unattractive look miserable? Are you exaggerating the importance of physical attractiveness for achieving life satisfaction? If unattractive people are living satisfied lives, why can't you as well?
"I can only live in misery and despair because of this chronic medical condition."	Talk to people you know with your medical condition, or read about people with this condition, or join a support group. Take note of how other people live with this condition. Is it true that having the condition automatically produces misery and despair? Are there people with it who are living more contented lives at this moment?

It will take some imagination and creativity on your part to think of activities you can schedule that will challenge your negative automatic thoughts and reinforce the more balanced, realistic alternative thoughts. However, the more you actually act on the alternative ways of thinking, the more natural they will become, and the fainter the voice of your harsh inner critic will become.

Facing the Challenge

No doubt you've heard the saying "There are three things that matter when you're selling property: location, location, location." The same could be said of cognitive mood repair, only we would say, " . . . practice, practice, practice." When you first start challenging your negative thinking with evidence gathering, error identification, generating alternatives, cost/benefit analysis, and taking action, you may find the whole process difficult and unnatural. But if you stick with it and practice these skills, you will get much better and more efficient. The process will begin to feel more natural, and as this happens, the power of these mood repair efforts will become more evident in your daily living. Psychologists and other mental health professionals have found these cognitive mood repair strategies to be some of the most powerful treatment interventions for overcoming daily sadness in people experiencing recurrent episodes of clinical depression.

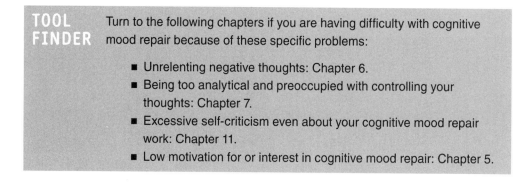

TOOL FINDER Turn to the following chapters if you are having difficulty with cognitive mood repair because of these specific problems:

- Unrelenting negative thoughts: Chapter 6.
- Being too analytical and preoccupied with controlling your thoughts: Chapter 7.
- Excessive self-criticism even about your cognitive mood repair work: Chapter 11.
- Low motivation for or interest in cognitive mood repair: Chapter 5.

5 take time to recharge

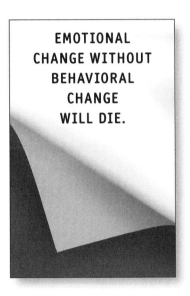

EMOTIONAL CHANGE WITHOUT BEHAVIORAL CHANGE WILL DIE.

Michelle, a 32-year-old mother of two children ages 7 and 5, was a full-time homemaker who exclaimed at her first therapy session, "I feel so tired and exhausted most of the time; I've lost all interest and motivation to do anything." She explained that for the first couple of years she'd enjoyed being at home with the children, involving herself throughout the day with child care, housework, and volunteer activities. In the last 3 years, however, she had been feeling really low more and more often, especially on weekday afternoons.

When asked about her mood, Michelle kept referring to her lack of energy and motivation and the fact that she couldn't get anything done. Normally a highly active person who could easily multitask, she was dismayed with how "lazy" she had become. When she felt sad, she also would feel overcome by a wave of fatigue and would end up sitting in the family room, mindlessly watching afternoon talk shows. Although she was tired, she could not sleep. Michelle was barely able to meet the demands of her 5-year-old, who arrived home from kindergarten at 2:30. During these times Michelle loathed herself, feeling intense guilt for just lying around the house. She isolated herself from others, and her husband learned not to call home in the afternoons because Michelle would rarely pick up the phone. Michelle felt as if there was no way out of her predicament.

Our behavior automatically changes when we feel depressed. We tend to withdraw from others and reduce our involvement in life, as if to conserve our energy. Michelle realized she should get up and do something, but she couldn't seem to push herself off the couch. And yet the more she rested, the more drained she felt.

Psychologists have learned that changing behavior is the best way to overcome the loss of energy and motivation people experience during bouts of dysphoria. In fact, one psychological intervention for clinical depression is called *behavioral activation*, and it has been shown to be a highly effective treatment.[1] This chapter presents the key strategies used in behavioral activation, and shows how you can use these strategies to overcome the loss of interest and motivation you feel during periods of low mood.

> It's a paradox: Activity is the best way to counteract the fatigue that makes you feel you can't do anything when your mood is low.

Use behavioral mood repair when you . . .

- feel depressed and notice a loss of interest or enjoyment.
- lack energy or must expend much greater effort than usual to do even ordinary activities.
- engage in extensive avoidance, withdrawal, or isolation during your blue periods.
- experience repeated bouts of depressed mood, despite using the situational and cognitive mood repair strategies described earlier in this book.

Changing how you behave can have a profound impact on how you feel, because there is a strong connection among thoughts, feelings, and behavior. Take a look at the diagram below.

Reducing your positive behaviors, and avoiding tasks and activities, both increase your negative thinking about yourself and your life situation. Michelle would watch TV for hours, all the time having negative thoughts about guilt and shame. As Chapter 4 has explained, negative thoughts can easily lead to depressed mood. So can reduced behavior. The two together have even more powerful depressive effects. *This is why it is important to include a combination of cognitive and behavioral mood repair strategies in your efforts to overcome depressed mood.*

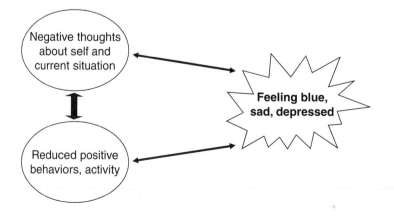

➤➤➤ Repair Strategy **17**:
Complete a Behavioral Inventory

To get the most from behavioral mood repair, it is important to find your baseline—that is, to learn about the nature of your current activity level and to determine how much you are accomplishing even when you are feeling depressed. People who get absolutely no sense of accomplishment or pleasure in anything they do during the day are rare indeed.

Use Repair Strategy 17 when you . . .

- can't figure out what makes you feel pleasure or mastery.
- can't seem to get yourself moving because you don't know what to do.

If you completed the Hourly Emotion Record in Chapter 2 (Repair Strategy 2), you may find it helpful to begin by reviewing the daily activities you recorded that were associated with higher ratings of happiness and lower ratings of sadness. These are the activities you will want to target for use in behavioral mood repair. Whether or not you completed the Hourly Emotion Record, the current strategy involves using a more specific self-monitoring form for behavioral change—a form that involves rating the sense of accomplishment and enjoyment you got out of your daily activities. So you should also complete a behavioral inventory using this new form, the Hourly Behavior Record, even if you kept an Hourly Emotion Record earlier.

REPAIR STRATEGY 17 INSTRUCTIONS

1. **On a sheet of paper, create a form based on the partial Hourly Behavior Record shown on the next page, or print out a complete one from *www.guilford.com/ clark7-forms*.** Plan to complete this form over a 1- to 2-week period, so that you will obtain a good sample of your daily behavior.

2. **Write down a short phrase that describes your main activity or behavior during each hour. It should take you just a few seconds to make this entry at the top of the hour.** If you forget to record an hour or two, leave it blank. It's important to make sure you complete the form close to the time of the activity, rather than relying on memory, which will not give you an accurate account of your behavior.

3. **When you enter the activity or behavior, also rate the degree to which it was associated with a sense of accomplishment or mastery, and the degree of enjoyment or pleasure it gave you. Make both ratings on a 0–10 scale, where 0 =**

Hourly Behavior Record

Hour	Main activity or behavior (during past hour)	Accomplish-ment (0–10)	Enjoyment (0–10)
5:00 A.M.			
6:00 A.M.			
7:00 A.M.			
8:00 A.M.			
9:00 A.M.			

absolutely no sense of accomplishment or enjoyment, 5 = considerable accomplishment/enjoyment, and 10 = extreme accomplishment/enjoyment.

4. **Once you've completed the Hourly Behavior Record for a week or two, review your entries and look for key behavioral trends that might be contributing to your depressed mood.** Are certain behaviors or activities that occur repeatedly associated with low ratings of accomplishment or enjoyment? Circle these behaviors and then compare them with the Hourly Emotion Record. Are these negative behaviors occurring at times when you feel more depressed? Could they be contributing to your depression? Highlight the behaviors you need to reduce to repair depressed mood.

5. **Now return to the Hourly Behavior Record and review it for activities or behaviors associated with high ratings of accomplishment and/or enjoyment. Put an asterisk beside each of these.** Again, compare these positive behaviors with your Hourly Emotion Record, and see whether they are associated with happier, more joyful mood. If so, these are the behaviors you may want to increase to improve your mood.

6. **Now record the positive behaviors from step 5 and the negative behaviors from step 4 in separate columns on another sheet of paper, so you can refer to it and make an effort to maximize positive and minimize negative activities. Save this list to use in Repair Strategy 18.**

Michelle's Hourly Behavior Record revealed a number of things she was doing that contributed to her depressed mood. She discovered that she was watching TV for 1–4 hours practically every afternoon during the week, and yet she rated it only a 2 for enjoyment and 0 for accomplishment. Other activities, like doing laundry and picking up after the children, were also associated with ratings of low accomplishment (3/10) and no enjoyment (0/10). Michelle noticed from her Hourly Emotion Record that these were times when she felt most depressed. Although watching afternoon TV, doing laundry, and tidying up were clearly negative behaviors that contributed to Michelle's depressed mood, the alternative was different for each activity. Reducing the amount of TV watching was an obvious solution for that depressive behavior, but doing laundry and picking up after the children were necessary household tasks she could not avoid. Therefore, the solution for those behaviors had to be different.

Michelle identified several positive behaviors from her Hourly Behavior Record that were associated with a higher sense of accomplishment or enjoyment. For example, talking to her sister on the phone and engaging with others on social media, especially Facebook, were rated as highly enjoyable (8/10). Also, having a cup of coffee in the morning and reading the newspaper gave her a heightened sense of accomplishment (7/10) and enjoyment (8/10), because she felt that she was keeping in touch with the outside world. When she compared the Hourly Behavior and Emotion Records, she noticed that her positive mood was rated higher when she engaged in these activities.

> Even minor daily tasks can lead to a greater sense of enjoyment or mastery that will lift your spirits.

What Can You Do If You Can't Stand the Boredom?

As a university professor, I work with young people on a daily basis. Many of my students complain about boredom, whether it's during a class, while studying, or on Sundays. It's as if boredom were the most excruciating state possible, to be avoided at all costs. (That's why it's better to text your friends than listen to a "boring lecture"!) But there is a problem with this complaint: Namely, much of what we must do in this life is boring. We can't be engaged and excited all the time, so we have to learn to tolerate the state of being bored.

Do you have problems with tolerating boredom? Do you find that you feel more depressed while doing a boring task? If you know you're about to engage in such a task, you can prepare yourself and reduce its negative effects on your mood. Review your Hourly Behavior Record, and highlight the daily tasks associated with low accomplishment or enjoyment. It may be that you can't avoid these tasks—but you can pre-pare yourself mentally to tolerate the routine, the mundane, or the boring (housecleaning, paying bills, mowing the lawn, etc.). In fact, even reminding yourself that a task is going to be tedious, unpleasant, or mundane but time-limited can reduce its effects on your depressed mood (e.g., "I can get through this and get on to something more enjoyable or rewarding").

Let me mention one other possibility about mundane, boring tasks. You might discover the "joy of boredom" in some of these routine activities. Sometimes daily tasks can be a diversion and offer some relaxation and respite from more demanding work. Recently I rediscovered an ancient mundane task—splitting firewood by hand (i.e., using an axe rather than a motorized wood-splitter). It's a really boring, repetitive task, but taking a half-hour break from writing to split wood is a great diversion for me. So maybe you too could turn some of the low-enjoyment/low-accomplishment tasks on your Hourly Behavior Record into a diversion, a "joy of boredom" activity. Why not give it a try?

> **Increase your tolerance, and even enjoyment, of daily living's routine, mundane tasks.**

TOOL FINDER Chapter 13 offers more discussion on dealing with the necessary but unrewarding tasks of life.

⤐ Repair Strategy ⓲: Invigorate Your Behavioral Inventory

You may notice from your review of your Hourly Behavior Record that you engage in few positive activities that bring you enjoyment or a sense of accomplishment. Maybe you've been struggling with the blues for such a long time that there is little joy or contentment in your life.

Use Repair Strategy 18 when . . .

- there is a low level of pleasure or mastery in almost all your daily living activities.

- your daily functioning is minimal, as indicated by a dramatic reduction in your activity level.

- you've become dependent on others to look after your tasks of daily living.

REPAIR STRATEGY 18 INSTRUCTIONS

1. **Take the two-column list of positive and negative behaviors you completed at the end of Repair Strategy 17. Assign a difficulty rating to increasing the frequency of the positive behaviors and reducing the frequency of the nega-tive behaviors, using a 10-point rating scale (0 = no difficulty, 5 = moderate difficulty, 10 = extreme difficulty). Enter the ratings on the list next to each behavior.** Michelle, for example, felt that spending more time on Facebook would actually be quite easy to do (1/10 difficulty rating), but that reducing the amount of TV watching would be harder (6/10 difficulty rating).

2. **Next, try to increase your list of positive behaviors by thinking back to the kinds of things you used to do in the past that brought you some enjoyment.** Do some brainstorming: What past hobbies, leisure activities, recreation, sports, or socializing did you enjoy in the past, even possibly years ago? You could ask your spouse/partner, a close friend, or a family member to help you remember past pleasurable or rewarding activities that you have long since stopped doing. Add these past pleasures to your positive behavior list, and give each one a difficulty rating (i.e., a rating of how hard it would be to start doing this activity).

3. **Now think about any new behaviors you could add to your inventory that might bring you a sense of accomplishment. Add those, and rate the difficulty of includ-ing them in your routine.** If you are having trouble thinking of pleasure/mastery behaviors, you can find several lists of these on the Internet by searching for "pleas-ant events list" (e.g., *www.healthnetsolutions.com/dsp/PleasantEventsSchedule.pdf*). You will find that these lists include a wide range of behaviors, from very simple things (like lighting a candle) to more complex, expensive activities (such as taking a cruise). Pick out a few activities from such a list that might be of interest or relevance to you, and add them to your inventory. It may be that going through a standard list will help you come up with additional ideas for positive behaviors.

4. **Now do the same for negative activities: Brainstorm negative behaviors that occur when you're in a depressed mood and that are associated with low lev-els of enjoyment or accomplishment.** These might include eating junk food, sleeping, watching TV, complaining, yelling at your children, arguing with your spouse/partner, driving more aggressively, avoiding work, isolating yourself from others, avoiding conversations, or surfing the Internet. As noted earlier, some-times behaviors that seem pleasurable leave you with a low sense of accomplish-ment (eating junk food might be an example), so it can be tricky to make this determination. Often activities that feel good momentarily but leave you feeling lousy are behaviors associated with low motivation and may occur naturally as attempts to conserve your energy. The problem is that these turn out to be poor

coping responses that actually worsen your depressed feelings in the long run. Avoidance is also often at the heart of these depressive behaviors. So it's important to identify these behaviors, giving each a rating of how difficult it would be to reduce the behavior. Again, you could ask your spouse/partner or a close friend what this person sees you doing when you're in a depressed mood. Your list of negative behaviors will probably be shorter than the positive behavior list, but no less important to change when it comes to mood repair.

5. **Finally, rank your two lists of positive and negative behaviors from the least difficult to change to the most difficult to change. Also, take a look at the enjoyment/ accomplishment ratings associated with the positive behaviors and the sadness ratings associated with the negative behaviors. Circle the positive behaviors that are less difficult to change but associated with significant enjoyment/accomplishment, and work on increasing these behaviors in your daily life. Do the same for the negative behaviors: Circle the ones that are less difficult to change but associated with a moderate level of sadness, and begin to work on reducing these behaviors in your daily living.** You will find Repair Strategy 20 particularly useful for reducing negative behavior, and Repair Strategy 21 for increasing positive behaviors.

⟫⟫→ Repair Strategy ⓭:
Set Goals for Behavioral Change

By now you may have started your behavioral mood repair work. After completing the previous two strategies, you may have developed a good understanding of the behaviors you need to increase and others you need to decrease to repair your depressed mood. You may even have made enough behavioral changes to make a noticeable difference in your negative mood. But if not, you may have lacked inspiration because you weren't targeting the areas of life that are most important to you. Repair Strategy 19 can be skipped if you are already increasing positive behaviors and reducing negative activities. However, if you are feeling stuck, try working through this goal-setting task, although you will need to do the work in Repair Strategies 17 and 18 first.

Use Repair Strategy 19 as a supplementary mood repair strategy when . . .

- you're not sure where to begin with making behavioral changes in your daily living.
- you've made some changes in your activity level, but you don't see any impact on your mood state.
- you have significant reservations or doubts about the importance of behavioral change in daily living.

REPAIR STRATEGY 19 INSTRUCTIONS

1. **Start by setting some priorities. How would you like to change? In terms of what is important to you—your personal values and goals in life—what are the most significant, meaningful tasks that you would like to target for change?** Making behavioral changes in the important areas of your life will have the greatest impact on repairing your depressed mood. So what life goals are most important to you: family relations, marriage, work, finances, recreation, health, leisure, friendships, spiritual matters . . . ? Select one or two of these areas as a guide for your behavioral change program. Write those areas down on a piece of paper.

2. **Now think about what positive behaviors you could increase and what negative behaviors you could decrease to improve each of those life areas.** For example, let's assume that one of the important goals or values in your life is financial independence. Maybe you grew up in a family where this was emphasized, or you've had some life experiences that make you concerned about debt, income, and spending. You might discover that positive behaviors such as putting a portion of your income into savings, paying off credit card balances, and taking public transit to work are associated with a sense of accomplishment, because they are connected with your goal of financial independence. At the same time, certain negative behaviors such as being late on bill payment, spending a lot of money on alcohol and cigarettes, and ordering takeout food for practically every meal may all be associated with feeling more depressed. It would be important to target these behaviors, because they undermine your goal of financial independence.

3. **Now begin your behavioral change program by targeting goal-related behaviors. Increase behaviors that move you closer to attaining your goal, and decrease behaviors that thwart goal attainment.**

4. **When you are feeling down or blue, determine whether you are engaging in negative, goal-interfering behavior. If so, work on replacing that behavior with positive, goal-enhancing behavior.** In our example, let's say that you notice feeling more depressed after eating takeout food on a weeknight, even though you maintain a healthy diet and weight range. What bothers you is the waste of money associated with this behavior. So now you know through the goal-setting task that coming home from work, feeling down and depressed, and actually spending the extra time to prepare a home-cooked meal will improve your mood, because it will feel to you like you're doing the responsible thing.

As Michelle reviewed her Hourly Behavior Record and list of positive and negative behaviors, she ranked improving her relationships with her children and husband as a high-priority goal. She then examined the positive behaviors she would need to increase (asking the children about their day at school, sitting with them during their after-school snack, etc.) and the negative behaviors she would need to decrease (refraining from yelling at the children for being messy, stopping the self-deprecating rants to her husband that she was fat and lazy, etc.) to reach this goal.

For her goal, Mai Lee wanted to be less stressed at work, which she associated with increased depressed mood. To achieve this, she realized she needed to stop arriving at work late, staying late to catch up, and feeling rushed and impatient in commuter traffic. At the same time, she needed to limit the amount of time she socialized with her coworkers (which she enjoyed but which kept her behind in her work), start work on projects earlier rather than procrastinate, and be more assertive with her supervisor about her workload.

> **Set specific goals for behavioral change.**

⫸⫸⫸ Repair Strategy ㉒: Embrace Behavioral Change

Even if the preceding strategies have already helped you make important behavior changes, certain behaviors may be proving especially resistant.

Use Repair Strategy 20 when . . .

- certain negative behaviors are proving especially difficult to change.
- a negative behavioral pattern has a strong impact on your mood.
- the negative behavior is a long-standing problem; you've made some behavioral changes, but more change is needed to make a real difference in your mood state.
- you want to prevent a return of the blues.

The centerpiece of the behavioral activation approach involves a framework for change that goes by the acronym ACTION and is the focus of this strategy:[1]

A = Assess mood and behavior.

C = Choose alternative behaviors.

T = Try out the alternative.

I = Integrate the changes into your life.

O = Observe the results.

N = Now evaluate.

REPAIR STRATEGY 20 INSTRUCTIONS

1. <u>A</u>ssess: **Review your Hourly Behavior Record (Repair Strategy 17), difficulty ratings (Repair Strategy 18), and goal-setting work if you did it (Repair Strategy 19) to select a negative or maladaptive behavior that occurs during your depressed moods, is associated with low enjoyment or achievement, interferes in an important goal, and is not too difficult to change.** You will want to take ACTION on a variety of maladaptive behaviors that contribute to depressed mood, so it is best to be strategic. Start with behaviors that are less difficult to change, and work your way up to the most difficult maladaptive behaviors.

   Michelle selected "yelling at the children for creating a mess" as a negative behavior that only made her feel more irritated and depressed, because the kids wouldn't listen; they would only become more defiant, and so she would start "nagging," as she put it. This was definitely undermining her desire for a better relationship with her children, and since this "nagging" behavior was rather recent, she thought that it wouldn't be too difficult to change. Later she tackled her excessive afternoon TV watching, which she thought would be more difficult to change, because she had always struggled with excessive TV viewing. Her initial attempts to change both behaviors had met with little success, so she realized she needed to use the more intense, focused ACTION strategy.

2. <u>C</u>hoose: **Think of an alternative behavior that is incompatible with the negative behavior you are trying to eliminate.**

   Michelle thought about her "nagging" behavior and about how else she could deal with the problem of messy children. She talked to her husband and a couple of other mothers about the problem, and even consulted a couple of books on parenting. The alternative she developed was to hold a family meeting and tell the kids that a messy house really bothered her, but she didn't like nagging at them all the time, so she was asking them not to make a mess in the room she was working in. She realized it was unreasonable to expect the kids not to make a mess in the room they were playing in, so 15 minutes before bedtime, the children and parents would tidy up the house together. In return, Michelle promised to stop nagging the children about the mess around the house. Everyone at the family meeting agreed to this new plan. Michelle actually made a game of it by drawing up an agreement that everyone then signed, and she posted this on the refrigerator door as a reminder. To help curb her tendency to nag, the children were given permission to remind their mother of the agreement whenever Michelle complained about a mess.

   Some alternative behaviors may call for a problem-solving approach, as in the previous example. Other alternative behaviors may involve doing something that is more pleasurable or gives you a greater sense of accomplishment. Eric often fell asleep for at least an hour after having a beer when he got home from work, and then he would wake up feeling hungry, irritated, and gloomy. The naps made it hard to fall asleep later and thus harder to get up in the morning, which in turn made him more depressed and interfered with his work performance. As an alternative, Eric decided to schedule some form of regular exercise right after work with a friend who was physically active. He used to enjoy squash, biking, and even brisk walking, so he decided to focus on these high-pleasure/high-mastery activities that he had listed when expanding his positive activities list in Repair Strategy 18. By reducing a negative behavior and adding a positive one, Eric doubled the benefits he got from this strategy.

> **TOOL FINDER**   Chapter 12 provides strategies that take advantage of exercise's ability to repair mood all by itself.

The alternative behavior with the greatest depressive mood repair capabilities will have the following characteristics:

- It will provide a more balanced, adaptive solution to a problem situation.

- It will lead to eliminating, or at least reducing, the maladaptive behavior.

- It will be more enjoyable, more rewarding, or associated with a greater sense of accomplishment.

3. <u>Try</u>: **Plan to engage in the alternative behavior for a defined period of time. You will need to be specific about the new behavior or activity, by writing down exactly what you will do, when, where, and with whom.** It can be very hard to change a routine and try something new. At first it won't feel right, and you may not notice an immediate improvement in your depressed mood. But intentionally schedule it into your day, and give the new behavior enough time to have an effect on how you feel. Strengthen your commitment to try the alternative by telling your spouse/partner or a close friend about your plan. Having an "accountability partner" is a great way to increase motivation for change.

> Alternative coping that is incompatible with avoidance has the greatest mood repair effect.

Michelle announced her "anti-nagging" plan to her family, and Eric involved a friend in his after-work exercise program.

4. <u>I</u>ntegrate: Repeatedly engage in the new behaviors over several days, trying to work them into your daily routine. New ways of behaving that fit more naturally into your daily routine have a greater chance of being maintained over time. If, for example, you're trying to be friendlier with coworkers, greeting them when you first get to work may fit better with the flow of office activity than trying to do it later, when everyone is busy. Also, it will take practice before the new behavior feels more natural and takes less effort. Let's say that you're trying to reduce your Internet surfing in the evening by reading novels; this will not have a big impact on your mood if you do it only once or twice. Instead, it has to be done repeatedly and become part of your daily routine before you'll notice any positive effects on your mood.

5. <u>O</u>bserve and <u>N</u>ow evaluate: Take special notice of the effects of the behavioral change on your level of happiness and sadness. Use the 10-point scale to rate your momentary level of happiness and sadness after executing the alternative behavior. Now compare this to the mood ratings for the same time of day written in your Hourly Emotion Record. Is the alternative behavior associated with an increase in positive mood and a decrease in negative mood? Do you need to make any changes in the behavior that would improve its mood repair impact? Has the alternative behavior resulted in a reduction of the maladaptive behavior that contributed to sadness? If the effects of this behavioral change have been positive, how long did they last?

   Michelle tried out her anti-nagging strategy over 2 weeks. At first she found it hard to ignore the children's mess, but over time it became easier. She noticed that the children reduced their sauciness toward her and were actually more cooperative in picking up before bedtime. More important, she felt less irritable and was better able to focus on getting more things done around the house after school. After getting positive feedback from her husband, she decided to stick with her program. She then moved on to tackle a more difficult maladaptive behavior—her excessive TV viewing in the afternoon.

⟫⟫⟫➤ Repair Strategy ㉑: Boost Rewarding Behavior

At this point, you should be both decreasing negative behavior and increasing positive behavior. However, many people struggling with the blues focus more on eliminating the negative, because when they are down they don't expect that their efforts to experience joy or satisfaction will succeed, and they convince themselves that trying is too hard. So they avoid exposing themselves to the very experiences that can improve their mood state. Therefore, this strategy is a specific focus on increasing the extent of rewarding or reinforcing experiences in your daily living.

Use Repair Strategy 21 when . . .

- you have been working especially hard at eliminating negative behavior and have neglected to work on enjoyment and rewarding activities.

- you can't remember the last time you enjoyed anything or felt happy.

- you have difficulty even thinking about your daily experiences in terms of level of joy, contentment, satisfaction, or accomplishment.

REPAIR STRATEGY 21 INSTRUCTIONS

1. **Start by looking back over your Hourly Behavior Record (Repair Strategy 17) and your list of past positive behaviors or activities (Repair Strategy 18). Now write down a list of activities associated with at least a moderate degree of enjoyment or sense of accomplishment—a rating of 5 or above.** In an average week, how much of your time is devoted to moderately enjoyable or rewarding activities? Are there particular times of the day when you are least likely to have positive experiences? Do these times of low-pleasure/low-mastery activities also coincide with depressed mood? If positive experiences occupy less than one-third of your time, you probably suffer from a low rate of positive reinforcement. Addressing this imbalance can have a significant mood repair effect.

2. **Select several moderately enjoyable or rewarding behaviors from your list, and start scheduling these activities into your day.** Try to schedule them during times of low mood. Also incorporate a variety of behaviors or activities that vary in time and complexity—from very simple, quick activities (like taking a warm bath, savoring a fresh cup of coffee, or checking your Facebook page) to the more complex (like taking a walk in the park, having dinner with a friend, or gardening). Some activities should simply provide pleasure; others should give you a sense of accomplishment, such as cleaning up a corner of the basement or signing up for a beginning art class. And some should introduce something new to your life, since novelty almost always boosts mood.

3. **Observe and evaluate the effects of injecting more rewarding and enjoyable experiences in your daily living.** What impact are your new efforts having on the blues? Are you letting yourself fully experience the little pleasures of life? The little pleasures of life aren't intended to "cure" sadness—but they can make small repairs in mood by taking you out of your negative thoughts and feelings momentarily, and helping you focus on the positive aspects of *this* moment.

TOOL FINDER   Chapter 7 offers strategies for staying in the present, which can help you avoid the ruminating and rehashing that fuel negative thoughts and emotions.

Michelle realized that she needed to be much more proactive about the slump she felt every afternoon. So she reviewed her Hourly Behavior Record and list of positive and negative activities, and came up with a variety of more pleasurable and rewarding activities she could do between noon and 4:00 P.M. She decided to have lunch out with a friend at least once a week; she joined a book club that met in the early afternoon; she signed up for an exercise class at the local gym; and she devoted some time each day to planning and then implementing a new gardening project. She also shifted some of her enjoyable self-care activities, such as hair appointments and facials, from mornings to afternoons. By systematically and intentionally building more pleasure and mastery activities into the more depressing part of her day, Michelle was able to make major gains in getting herself out of the afternoon slump.

▶ Repair Strategy ㉒: Savor the Change

Behavior change provides its own rewards, but you can intensify its mood repair effects by recognizing and celebrating the work you've done and the accomplishments you've made. Take time to stand back, reflect on the positive effects of your behavioral changes, and consider how you've taken control of your emotional state.

A couple of years ago, I built a 12- by 12-foot cedar gazebo for my daughter's wedding. It was a very challenging project that took several months to complete, in part because it had to be built on a steep riverbank. To this day, I sit in the gazebo, reflect on the construction, and feel a great deal of satisfaction with its accomplishment. I could sit in the gazebo and look at all the mistakes I made (and there were plenty), or I could sit and think about the accomplishment. Alternatively, I could ignore the gazebo altogether and focus my attention on another project. By taking time and choosing to reflect on my accomplishment, I experience a positive feeling of mastery and high satisfaction. If you've been feeling overwhelmed by the blues, get a little relief by focusing on progress or positive changes you've made recently.

REPAIR STRATEGY 22 INSTRUCTIONS

1. **Take time out from planning your next change effort to review the work you've already done successfully.** At this point you may be tempted to focus on

the behavioral changes you still need to make, and in fact more change may be needed. Still, shift your focus to what you've accomplished. There will be plenty of time later to deal with additional changes.

2. **Practice expressions of self-congratulation.** Most people find it hard to admit that they've accomplished something or done a good job. It's hard enough to accept the praise of others, but it may seem downright immoral to praise oneself. And yet some degree of self-praise is important for maintaining behavioral change. If you are trying to quit smoking, for example, you need to praise yourself when you have small victories, or you'll quickly give up. The same will happen with your efforts to engage in behavioral mood repair: You'll give up and sink back into the blues if you don't recognize your accomplishments.

3. **Declare your progress to others.** As mentioned earlier, accountability to others is a significant motivator for behavioral change. (It is a big factor in the success of Alcoholics Anonymous and other Twelve-Step groups, notably.) So mention your intentions for behavioral change to family members and close friends, and update them on your progress with behavioral change. Telling them of your successes (e.g., "I went to the gym three times this week") will be more helpful in maintaining your behavioral changes than beating yourself up by telling them of your failures.

4. **Recite your successes when you become discouraged.** When you're feeling blue and filled with self-doubt, remind yourself of the behavioral changes you've made and your progress with mood repair. I'm not suggesting that you delude yourself by sugar-coating what you've achieved, but recognizing real success will reinforce your competence and keep you going when the going gets tough.

When Michelle was feeling discouraged, she could remind herself that she had cut down on the TV viewing and napping, and wasn't nagging the children as much. We all feel a momentary lift in our mood when we are reminded of successes, so why not use this strategy the next time you feel depressed or discouraged? You too should try to remember where you began and what has changed in your life since you started doing behavioral mood repair.

Barriers to Behavioral Change

If you've been trying behavioral change, has it lived up to your expectations? Maybe you've encountered a significant personal barrier to your efforts. For behavioral change to have a positive impact on your mood, the right attitude is absolutely critical. Remember the diagram earlier in this chapter, which shows the strong relationship between the way you think and the way you act. Is it possible that you've been beaten down by the blues so many times that deep down, you harbor a belief that you're helpless to fight your moods? In his book *Beat the Blues before They Beat You,* Robert Leahy has identified several negative thoughts and beliefs that characterize low motivation. Take a close look at these, and ask yourself honestly whether you subscribe to these ideas about yourself:

"I can't get myself to do anything."

"There is no sense in trying, because it won't help."

"I don't have the energy to do anything."

"I'll wait until I feel less depressed."

"I won't enjoy it, so why bother?"

"I'm just too lazy to do anything."

"I don't deserve to feel better."

"I can't do anything until I feel motivated."

"I need to want to do something before I can do it."

"It's all too overwhelming, so why even get started?"

"It's much better to do nothing and save my energy."

"I'll never succeed, so there's no sense in trying."

"I should be able to do this easily; it's discouraging that even the simplest tasks take so much out of me."

This type of thinking is not harmless. All these thoughts can lead to inaction and a profound sense of helplessness.

TOOL FINDER If a sense of helplessness is interfering in your ability to engage in behavioral mood repair, you'll find the cognitive repair techniques in Chapter 4 particularly valuable. In fact, these may be essential before you can fully succeed at behavior change.

The Power of Change

As noted in earlier chapters, cognitive behavior therapy is known to be one of the most effective treatments for clinical depression. Change in both negative thoughts (see Chapter 4) and mood-lowering behaviors (this chapter) is considered critical to the treatment. *That's why the strategies in these two chapters serve as the foundation of all the other mood repair strategies discussed in this book.* You may want to bookmark these chapters and return to them frequently as you incorporate other interventions into your mood repair toolkit.

6 stop the mental treadmill

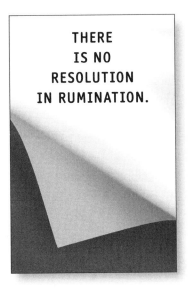

**THERE
IS NO
RESOLUTION
IN RUMINATION.**

You're probably familiar with how a treadmill works: It goes around and around, and anyone or anything on it—you at the gym, or a hamster in a cage—gets a physical workout but doesn't actually go anywhere. Of course, the whole point of a treadmill is that you expend a great deal of energy and end your workout feeling exhausted, but you haven't actually changed your location. You wind up exactly where you started, in the same room, staring at the same TV monitor. To be honest, that's one reason I prefer running outdoors: At least when you're outside, you're going somewhere. The distance gives the illusion that you're making progress, even though you end up back where you started.

Some people who get stuck in the blues end up on a "mental treadmill." In the same way that an exercise treadmill can wear you out (in a good way), on a mental treadmill you can run yourself ragged (in a bad way) and never leave your present location. You get caught in a vicious cycle of thinking—a type of negative self-reflection that churns away over and over in an uncontrollable and unproductive manner. This mental treadmill experience is called *rumination,* and it's the topic of this chapter. Some researchers believe that rumination is an important contributor to turning normal sadness or distress into clinical depression.[1]

Rumination can turn depressed mood into clinical depression.

Harold, a 43-year-old married plumber, decided it was time to see a psychologist after suffering a severe episode of depression that was not responding well to antidepressant medication. Harold arrived at my office in a highly distressed, agitated state. He could hardly sit still in his chair; he fidgeted about and wrung his hands nervously. As we talked, one symptom stood out above the low mood, lack of motivation, fatigue, and insomnia that confirmed his clinical depression: *depressive rumination.* During the course of the interview, Harold kept saying things like "I'm so depressed. What am I going to do? I shouldn't be depressed; I have no right to be depressed. I'll never get out of this depression, so what am I going to do?" Although Harold was able to talk about other aspects of his problem, he returned again and again to these themes of self-blame and catastrophic thinking about being depressed.

Over the course of our sessions, I learned that Harold had always been a serious, somewhat anxious individual, who could easily worry and become preoccupied with life's challenges. He was meticulous, if not rigid, stubborn, and perfectionistic, in his work and family relations. Harold was conscientious at work and a loyal and dedicated family man at home, but people found him intense, humorless, an "overthinker." The fact that he was also a moody person who could feel angry and frustrated with life, frequently falling deeply into the blues, made it even harder for others to be around him. Harold was also deeply religious, and his belief that "Christians should never be depressed" made it especially difficult for him to accept that he was losing his battle with the blues and needed professional help.

Harold became preoccupied with his diagnosis of clinical depression. He spent much of the day thinking over and over about how being depressed was the worst thing that could have happened to him, and how embarrassed he felt at being a person with depression. What would others think of him? Would he ever get better? How could God accept him for being defeated by depression? Harold also thought that depression was a sign of sin and lack of faith in God. He believed that if he prayerfully turned his problems over to God, his distress would disappear and he would feel peace and comfort, knowing he had a right relationship with God. The fact that he was highly distressed and agitated despite prayer meant to Harold that he did not have such a relationship. His ruminative thinking about the awfulness of his depression made his guilt and self-condemnation worse, pushing him into an extreme state of helplessness and hopelessness where he began to have suicidal thoughts. Harold's depressive rumination was a key reason not only for the persistence of his clinical depression, but possibly for its failure to respond to antidepressant medication.

> You cannot repair the blues while being preoccupied with how bad you feel or its negative impact on your life.

Rumination is a type of negative thinking that is passive but persistent and repetitive. An individual returns to the same themes over and over, "obsessing" about the depressive feelings, their causes, and their consequences.[1] It's a complicated process that involves different facets of thinking: unhelpful beliefs, emotion-focused ruminating, perfectionistic standards, and excessive self-criticism. Each of the four mood repair strategies presented in this chapter addresses one of these factors, although the last strategy is a more general intervention that can be used with all forms of depressive rumination.

It's important to note that although Harold was clinically depressed, rumination can affect anyone stuck in the blues. When such rumination is a habit, it can push sad mood into clinical depression, so it's important to address even if your problem doesn't seem as severe as Harold's.

TOOL FINDER Chapter 7 offers strategies based on mindfulness meditation, another useful approach to depressive rumination.

Depressive Rumination: The Mental Treadmill

As described above, Harold spent hours trying to understand why he became depressed, catastrophizing about being in that mood state, and berating himself for being such a bad Christian. This type of negative, repetitive thinking is the hallmark of rumination. Ruminating people can even get stuck on the same thought over and over:

"What's wrong with me?"

"Why can't I get over this depression?"

"What if I have to live this way the rest of my life?"

"What if the problem never goes away?"

"Why do I suffer these depressed moods more than others?"

Rumination is considered a passive form of thinking because it never leads anywhere. Harold's incessant thinking not only failed to resolve his mood, but actually made him a less productive worker who needed to take a medical leave and became more difficult to live with at home. But rumination can also be found in milder states of depressed mood. Tanisha, an 18-year-old, continually analyzed almost every interaction with peers; she was excessively concerned that they might not like her because she tended to be glum and was not very fun-loving. The fact is that you can ruminate on just about anything in your life, but in depressive rumination—the topic of this chapter—the person's repetitive thinking is about being distressed. So Tanisha ruminated about whether her friends liked her because she was often in a bad mood, whereas Josephine ruminated about not doing well in school because low grades made her feel depressed for several days.

Not only does depressive rumination lead nowhere; it actually cycles back onto itself. You start thinking about how bad it is to feel depressed, and you may think about various aspects of being depressed, but you always end up back at the beginning, which is how awful you feel when you're depressed.

In 30-plus years of working as a clinical psychologist, I have never met a person who found depressive rumination helpful. The research on this topic backs up this observation. Many negative effects are associated with depressive rumination. People who are prone to it also struggle with other forms of negative thinking, such as worry, pessimism, negative attitudes, and hopelessness. They often use less effective emotion coping strategies (like suppression and avoidance, discussed in Chapter 1). Furthermore, people who ruminate have a higher risk for clinical depression, and their depressions may last longer than those of people who become depressed but do not ruminate. In addition people who ruminate have longer and more intense periods of depressed mood, increased negativity about themselves and their life circumstances, lower motivation, reduced decision-making ability, less capacity to initiate productive activity, poorer social problem solving, and reduced social support.

The reason why rumination, as a way of thinking, leads to more depression is that it amplifies several psychological processes known to contribute to depression. These include dwelling on negative thinking and memories during depressed moods, engaging in poor problem solving, having reduced motivation, and experiencing less social support from others. Despite all the time he spent thinking about depression, Harold became more entrenched in his negativity. It seemed to interfere in his ability to make

> Rumination intensifies negative thinking, saps motivation, and interferes with problem solving.

decisions even about the simple things in life, such as whether to go somewhere in the afternoon or what to order at a restaurant. He was so stuck in his thoughts that he had little motivation to do anything, and people started avoiding him because all he talked about was how bad he felt. Given all the negative consequences associated with depressive rumination, it is important to eliminate this form of toxic negative thinking if it happens to you during times of feeling down.

Most of us become preoccupied with personal issues from time and time, and we may even be guilty of overthinking. Maybe at times you've even said to someone that you've been ruminating about such and such an issue. But after reading the previous description, you might be wondering whether your repetitive thinking is extreme enough to be considered depressive rumination. How can you know when your negative thinking has morphed into rumination? To help with this distinction, it is useful to know that psychologists also use the more specific term *brooding* to refer to a more toxic aspect of depressive rumination.

Brooding is a moody sort of pondering in which people focus on causal issues related to feeling depressed, such as "Why do I always react this way?" or "Why do I have problems other people don't have?" People who brood may often become immersed in self-blame, spending much time alone in critical self-examination.[1] A sense of gloom and anxiousness envelops them as their thinking becomes dominated by a negative comparison of their current situation with an unachieved outcome (e.g., "Why didn't I handle that situation better?"). Harold's brooding took the form of endlessly blaming depression on his lack of faith in God and his sinfulness, and then repeatedly asking himself why he didn't have more faith. His brooding led him to the conclusion that he could not possibly be a Christian, because he was depressed; therefore, he was condemned to hell.

Is your negative thinking depressive rumination? Check off any of the following descriptions that apply to you.

❏ You have been repeatedly having the same negative thoughts about yourself and your depressive mood state for several weeks or months.

❏ Your negative thinking is highly self-focused; others may even call it "self-pity."

❏ You are preoccupied with feeling depressed, which causes you to feel "depressed about being depressed."

❏ Your negative thinking feels stuck; you seem to be "thinking in circles."

❏ Your negative thinking feels out of control; you can't stop your mind from shifting into repetitive negative thinking.

❏ Your negative thinking is passive; it never leads to a solution or a more effective way to deal with your circumstances.

❏ You are an "overthinker"; your negative thinking becomes too deep, complicated, and abstract.

❏ Your negative thinking is highly self-critical in a vague, abstract, or generalized fashion ("Why am I such a loser?" or "Why does my life have no purpose or meaning?").

If you checked only one or two boxes, you are probably not ruminating (although this checklist is representative rather than exhaustive), and so you should skip the remainder of this chapter and proceed to Chapter 7. If you checked three or more boxes, it is likely that you engage in depressive rumination; definitely continue reading this chapter, in which I present five mood repair strategies you can use to reduce such rumination. Working with these strategies can shift your focus from brooding to acceptance, helpful action, and positive self-evaluation as pathways toward effective negative mood repair.

Use these strategies for reducing depressive rumination when...

- you meet at least three of the criteria in the preceding checklist.
- you've tried the cognitive repair strategies in Chapter 4, but your negative thinking persists.
- you feel as if you're "drowning" in the same pattern of negative thinking; you can't seem to think any other way about yourself or your negative mood state.
- people have tried to reason with you that your negative thinking is excessive, but it doesn't help.

⫸⫸ Repair Strategy ㉓: Complete a Rumination Impact Statement

People who struggle with depressive rumination often hold positive beliefs about their rumination, like these:

"To understand my feelings of depression, I need to think through my problems."

"I need to think repeatedly about my problems to find the causes of my depression."

"Thinking a lot about my problems helps me focus on the most important things."

"Dwelling on the past helps me prevent future mistakes and failures."

In fact, two British psychologists, Costas Papageorgiou and Adrian Wells, have found that these positive beliefs about rumination may actually *cause* people to ruminate.[2] In view of the ample evidence that rumination leads nowhere, it's amazing that people keep trying it. The way in which positive beliefs contribute to depressive rumination isn't well understood. Many people, like Harold, hold on to positive beliefs about rumination (Harold believed he had to continue to "work out his salvation"— that is, think through his terrible spiritual state through meditation and Biblical study), even though they recognize the harm it does. Harold was able to acknowledge that his endless preoccupation with depression was ruining his life—driving him further from his family and making it impossible to work productively. It is likely that once a person gets into the ruminative process, negative beliefs get activated and become more dominant, so the person becomes focused on the negative effects of the rumination. These negative beliefs—"Rumination makes me feel out of control, a bad person, a failure"—will then contribute to even stronger feelings of depression. So a person could start with the positive belief "If I think about this hard enough, I'll solve the problem," but end up with the negative conclusion "Why can't I solve this problem? I must be an idiot."

The power of erroneous positive beliefs about rumination is a compelling reason to start your battle against depressive rumination by challenging those beliefs, using the Rumination Impact Statement form presented on the next page.

> Contradictory positive and negative beliefs about rumination can coexist, with each contributing to the persistence of ruminative thinking.

If you have read Chapter 4, you're now familiar with the mood repair strategy called *cost/benefit analysis* (Repair Strategy 15). Completing a Rumination Impact Statement is very similar to doing a cost/benefit analysis to correct the negative thinking of depression, only this time it is focused specifically on the consequences of rumination.

Use Repair Strategy 23 when . . .

- you're uncertain about the impact of your ruminative thinking.

- you believe that thinking through your depression may have some benefits.

- you're not sure you're ready to change how you think when you're feeling depressed.

REPAIR STRATEGY 23 INSTRUCTIONS

1. **Identify the core issue or theme of your rumination.** Usually people ruminate about some aspect of feeling depressed, its causes, or its consequences. Harold, for example, ruminated on the inconsistency between his faith and his experience of depression ("Christians shouldn't get depressed"), as well as its consequences for his spiritual life ("God must have left me because I'm so depressed. Therefore, I'm condemned to eternal separation from God"). You may find that you ruminate about never getting over depression, not being able to sleep, lacking motivation or interest, losing some relationship, a strained marriage or family relationship, being less productive at work, or the like.

2. **Next, set aside 20–30 minutes when you are not feeling depressed, when you are alone, and when you won't be interrupted or rushed by life's demands. Take a sheet of paper and create two columns as illustrated in the partial Rumina-**

tion Impact Statement form below, or print out a complete form from *www. guilford.com/clark7-forms*.

3. **Begin by listing in the left column of the Rumination Impact Statement what you believe are the advantages—the possible benefits that may result from thinking over and over about some problem or aspect of feeling depressed.** What do you hope to achieve, or what have you achieved so far, from all this overthinking? Have you had any new insights, solved any life problems, or become stronger as a person through this repetitive thinking? Write down anything positive that has happened, or that you imagine or hope might happen, from ruminating about your current emotional state.

4. **Then, in the right column, write down all the negative consequences of rumination.** Has the repetitive thinking taken a toll on you? How has it affected your feelings and your behavior? Has rumination had any negative effects on your work performance, family relationships, physical health, and the like?

5. **Once you've completed both columns, go back and take a look at what you've written.** Is rumination worth it? Do the costs far outweigh any perceived benefits? What impact has rumination had on your life?

6. **Once you've completed and examined your Rumination Impact Statement, refer to it every time you start to ruminate. When you get stuck in depressive rumination, read over what you've written about your rumination, and add to the form any new insights you have about the rumination process.** You can use

Rumination Impact Statement

What I hope to achieve (benefits) by thinking over and over about this problem, or about my experience of feeling sad or blue	What negative effects (costs) are associated with thinking over and over about this problem, or about my experience of feeling sad or blue
1.	1.
2.	2.

the form to increase your motivation and resolve to deal with rumination in a more positive, adaptive manner.

Louise had two teenage sons she was finding very challenging to raise. She had frequent bouts of low mood during which she ruminated endlessly about her sons' defiance and rebelliousness, trying to figure out where she went wrong and why she was such a failure as a parent. This perceived failure was an important cause of Louise's descent into the blues. Following are the advantages and disadvantages Louise came up with for her depressive rumination.

Potential Benefits of Ruminating about Being a Bad Mother

"Maybe all this thinking will lead to some new insight about parenting teenage sons."

"Maybe all this thinking and worrying will motivate me to snap out of being depressed all the time."

"Maybe my husband will notice how upset I am getting, and will take more responsibility in disciplining our sons."

"Maybe my sons will see how upset I become, and will decide to be more cooperative."

"All this ruminating means I'm a sensitive, loving mother."

Potential Costs of Ruminating about Being a Bad Mother

"I notice that I'm having more frequent and longer bouts of depression since I started ruminating about the boys."

"My sons are spending less time at home; I feel like they are avoiding me when I get distressed."

"Since I am spending more and more time in my head about parenting and being depressed, I seem less able to communicate with my sons."

"I am having more arguments with my husband about parenting issues."

"Rumination is causing considerable strain on our marriage, because my husband tries to reason with me and talk me out of rumination, but it isn't helpful and so he just gets frustrated with me."

"When I ruminate at night, I can't get to sleep, and so I feel exhausted the next day."

"I think my parenting has actually gotten worse since I started ruminating, and so it's increased my conviction that I'm a bad mother."

"When I ruminate, I withdraw from other people, and so I've become more isolated from family and friends."

> Rumination may be taking a greater toll on your emotions than you realize.

"I don't get as much done around the house when I ruminate, and so I end up feeling lazy and useless."

Louise's Rumination Impact Statement challenged her preconceived beliefs that ruminating would help her find a better way to deal with her sons.

⟩⟩⟩➤ Repair Strategy ㉔: Reevaluate Your Depressive Mood

Earlier I have said that rumination tends to cycle back on itself, always bringing us back to repetitive thinking about how bad we're feeling because we're so down. This can be thought of as *emotion-focused rumination*, and it leaves us feeling "depressed about being depressed." Of course, being depressed about feeling the blues only intensifies negative thinking, which perpetuates the cycle between negative thoughts and negative emotions.

Louise, for example, would ruminate on what a failure she had been as a mother, which would then bring up reminders of all the other ways she had been a failure in life. This cycle of negative thinking made her even more aware of how depressed she had been feeling and how her bouts with depression made her such an ineffective parent. She could see no way out of her terrible situation as long as she was battling the blues. From Louise's perspective, being depressed was a major contributor to her parenting problem. Her ruminative periods became ever more focused on how terrible it was to be down and depressed so much of the time. Eventually Louise became convinced that her depressive moods were a major cause of her strained relationship with her sons, and that she was helpless to do anything about it. For Louise, having these dark and gloomy days became the most horrible affliction, which she believed was causing her life to spiral further downward uncontrollably.

The aim of this mood repair strategy is to address this biased, overly negative outlook on feeling depressed that so often occurs when people engage in depressive rumination. The central questions to ask yourself are these: "Is feeling sad really as bad as

I am making it out to be? What's so bad about having these bouts with the blues? How has low mood really affected my life?"

Use Repair Strategy 24 when . . .

- you find yourself ruminating on how bad you are feeling.

- you are feeling discouraged with your battle against the blues.

- you're trying to "think through" your depressive periods, but there seems to be no solution.

- you are worried about the effects of depression on your life.

REPAIR STRATEGY 24 INSTRUCTIONS

1. **Take a period of time when you are in a more positive (or at least neutral) mood, and write down an honest, fair, and realistic evaluation of the effects that negative mood or dysphoria has had on your life.** Try to stick to objective evidence of specific ways in which your sad mood episodes have affected you on a day-to-day basis. What tangible, actual events or outcomes are associated with feeling depressed? For example, how has low mood changed your work, family relations, physical health, relations with your spouse/partner, recreation, or social relations? Probably you can think of many negative ways sadness has affected your life, but what about potential positive effects? Has depressed mood made you a more sensitive, understanding, thoughtful person?

   Unless you are suffering from an episode of clinical depression that requires mental health treatment, it is likely that you are exaggerating the negative effects of "being in a funk." Most people, even when they are feeling down, still get their work done, interact with family and friends, keep up some form of recreation and relaxation, and so forth. In fact, even if you are clinically depressed, it is likely that you are doing a lot better than you think.

2. **During one of your sad mood episodes, try to capture on paper the main theme or content of your emotion-focused rumination.** How are you thinking about your experience with depression when you are ruminating about feeling down? What precisely about feeling blue is so upsetting for you? What terrible consequences are you thinking your moods will cause in your life? Are you blaming yourself, or trying to figure out the causes or solutions? If you completed the Rumination Impact Statement (Repair Strategy 23), you have already done a lot of this work. Review this form, but now write down on a separate sheet of paper a summary of the emotion-focused part of your rumination (how you ruminate about being depressed).

3. **Compare your more realistic, balanced appraisal of feeling down with your more negative, catastrophic view when you are engaged in depressive rumination.** What are the main differences between the two perspectives on being depressed? Focus on how your belief about feeling depressed becomes exaggerated when you ruminate. Which account of your experience of depression is more believable? As noted above, you should be doing this review when you are feeling less distressed, or at least are in a more neutral mood state. This way, the negativity that accompanies low mood is less likely to cloud your judgment.

4. **Whenever you experience depressive rumination that focuses on how bad you feel, take out your depression reevaluation summary and use it to correct any catastrophic thinking about being down that occurs when you are ruminating.** Use this reevaluation to remind yourself of all the ways in which depressed mood "is not as bad as I am thinking." This will help curb any mental hand wringing about being depressed; it will also help you develop a more accepting, less controlling approach to your negative mood episodes.

> **TOOL FINDER**   You'll find strategies for becoming more accepting of sadness in Chapter 7.

5. **If you are having difficulty generating a more realistic, balanced perspective on being down, ask someone close to you who has witnessed your periods of depression to help you with the task.** For example, your spouse or partner has probably seen you go through depressive mood episodes many times. What changes does he/she see in you when you're feeling blue? What are you able or not able to do during these episodes? Your spouse or partner can help you develop a more realistic perspective of the experience of feeling depressed, which you can then use to challenge your emotion-focused rumination.

As noted earlier, an important feature of Harold's rumination was his relentless preoccupation with the effects of depression on his spiritual well-being. A more realistic reevaluation of his depressed mood would reveal that he was not relinquishing as much of his faith as he thought. He was still going to church, still doing some Bible reading and prayer, and certainly still had a strong belief in God. His family, pastor, and church friends never wavered in their belief that Harold was a Christian. So the evidence indicated that depressed mood might not be having as devastating an impact on his spiritual life as he was thinking.

Also as noted previously, the emotion-focused part of Louise's rumination centered on the effects of depression on her parenting ability. Reevaluation of her dys-

> **Developing a realistic, balanced perspective on depressed mood is key to reining in your emotion-focused depressive rumination.**

phoric mood states revealed that she was still very much engaged in family life even when she was feeling sad; she did have moments of meaningful conversation with at least one son; she was still competent in how she managed the family finances; and she was still maintaining some contact with close friends. Louise concluded that her frequent bouts with the blues were having less of a negative impact than she thought.

TOOL FINDER   If you have strong beliefs about the negative effects of depressed mood, you can use the cognitive mood repair strategies in Chapter 4 to correct these beliefs.

➤➤➤ Repair Strategy 25: Recalibrate Your Standards

When we fail to achieve important life goals, we are more susceptible to ruminating about ourselves and our shortcomings. But sometimes we get trapped in this kind of thinking because our performance standards are too high or our social comparisons are too extreme. A colleague once told me of a scientist he treated who was depressed because he had failed to win a Nobel Prize—the pinnacle of scientific achievement—in his field of study. A woman I knew ended up clinically depressed because she could not lift herself out of the deep disappointment she felt about being "inferior" to all of her friends: She believed that she was not as wealthy, was not as attractive, had fewer accomplishments to her credit, had less successful children, lived in a smaller home, and had a husband who didn't appreciate her. Excessively high performance standards, perfectionism, and exaggerated upward social comparisons can all lead to a sense of failing to achieve important goals, and ultimately to more rumination and depressed mood. If you adhere to such standards, you may find yourself ruminating over why you've not succeeded, what you could do differently, why others seem to be doing so much better than you, and how bleak your future looks. Of course, this will lead not only to profound discontentment, but also to heightened negative mood.

One way to deal with this maladaptive form of comparison is to reevaluate your criteria for success. Maybe you are being more successful at goal achievement than you think, and the problem is that you have excessively high standards. When I was in junior high, I loved track and field, and I especially loved the high jump. But I was terrible at it because I was too short. I should have stuck to running, but instead I kept trying to compete in the high jump, and I kept failing. At the time, there was nothing more demoralizing than to watch everyone else clear a height that I repeatedly failed to jump. Maybe in your life you keep setting the bar too high, and so you repeatedly experience failure. Not everyone who experiences depressive rumination has excessively high standards, but if you do, this strategy will be helpful.

Use Repair Strategy 25 if . . .

- you have perfectionist tendencies.
- you often think about your failures, mistakes, and shortcomings when you are ruminating.
- others have said that your personal standards and expectations are too high.
- you often have a feeling of defeat.

REPAIR STRATEGY 25 INSTRUCTIONS

1. **Take a time when you are not feeling depressed, and make a list of your most important personal standards and expectations for yourself. Now evaluate these standards.** Given your history, life circumstances, talents, and abilities, are your goals too high? We all need moderately high goals to remain engaged and challenged in life pursuits, but are your goals excessive—or practically unattainable?

2. **Ask yourself some deeper questions about life.** Here are some examples:

   "What are my values and purposes in life?"

   "What do I want or think I need to reach this goal?"

   "Will I really feel better, happier, less depressed, and more contented if I reach this goal?"

   "In 10 or 20 years, will this goal seem so important?"

   "How do I want to be remembered?"

   "What do I really want to accomplish in life?"

3. **Discuss your goals, standards, and expectations with a close friend, a family member, or your therapist.** Do others consider your standards too high? How do your standards compare to those of others you know?

4. **During your ruminative periods, take out your standards and expectations list. Is evidence of these unrealistic goals and values creeping into your rumination?** If you find yourself thinking over and over again about failure, defeat, and disappointment, challenge your expectations and standards. How can you think about your accomplishments in a more realistic manner? Practice replacing an unattainable goal by rehearsing to yourself an alternative, more attainable standard.

> Keep in mind that your standards were not handed down from on high. You acquired them through life experiences, and so you can change them.

TOOL FINDER   Chapter 9 focuses specifically on goals, values, and personal standards. You will want to consult this chapter if perfectionism plays an important role in your struggle with depressive rumination.

▶▶▶ Repair Strategy ㉖: Schedule a Brooding Session

I have previously described *brooding* as a particularly toxic form of rumination in which you badger yourself about why your mood is low, your life is miserable, and you can't resolve either one. Obviously it often involves excessive self-blame and gloominess, which are particularly negative elements of depressive rumination.

One reason brooding may have such a strong link to depressive mood is that it seems so natural and yet uncontrollable. When you start ruminating in this way, it may seem spontaneous, as if it were the only thing you could do at the time. You don't have to remind yourself that it is time to start brooding; you seem to fall into it quite easily, unintentionally. Such spontaneous and automatic thinking seems more significant, more believable, and therefore more distressing. Imagine that you're sitting at home, it's late at night, and the thought suddenly pops into your head: "I wonder if my daughter is safe?" You may start worrying and feel yourself getting upset, because you assume that the thought popped into your head for a reason. "Maybe it means she really is in danger." On the other hand, if you are in my office and I ask you to think that your daughter is in danger, you could do it, but it would not be distressing. You would tell yourself it means nothing, because you are simply generating the thought "on demand"—making it up because I asked you to do it. When thought processes like brooding occur more naturally, out of the blue, the thoughts feel more "real" and more worthy of our attention. This gives us a clue on how to deal with ruminative brooding: If we strip brooding of its spontaneous, natural quality, it will become less distressing and more controllable.

Use Repair Strategy 26 when . . .

- you find yourself ruminating on why life has not gone the way you wished.
- you engage in a lot of self-blame and criticism.
- you do a lot of comparative thinking, in which you contrast your current situation with that of others or with some desired alternative outcome ("Why couldn't things be better?", "What did I do to deserve this?").
- your rumination causes you to feel more anxious and gloomy about the future.

REPAIR STRATEGY 26 INSTRUCTIONS

1. **Set aside 30–45 minutes each day for a self-imposed brooding session. Choose a time of day when you are not busy, and when you can find a quiet place to be alone and uninterrupted. Sit comfortably in a chair, close your eyes if it helps, and just let your mind wander to all the things you think about over and over when you're feeling depressed.** You want your intentional brooding session to be similar to natural, spontaneous brooding, so you want to make sure you're thinking about the same stuff as when you spontaneously start brooding.

2. **Your mind will wander during this session, so when you notice this happening, gently bring it back to your rumination issues.** Try to get yourself into a real "rumination stew"; that is, brood to the best of your ability. You can remind yourself that it's time to brood, so keep thinking over and over again: "Why don't I have any friends? What did I do to deserve my loneliness? Why don't people like me? Why do I feel so depressed? Why can't I get over it?" Just keep "whying" to yourself over and over. There's nothing to solve, so just keep asking why.

3. **You can use the Brooding Diary shown partially on the facing page (or print out a complete form from *www.guilford.com/clark7-forms*) to help you create the most effective rumination session.** When you start to fill in your Brooding Diary, think back to your struggles with rumination and ask yourself: "What do I think about when I ruminate? What issues do I keep thinking about over and over? What do I keep asking 'why' about?" People's memories are not very accurate and tend to be highly selective, so you will need to capture some real-life rumination

Brooding Diary

Thinking about causes for my sadness/situation	Thinking about how I am dealing with feeling sad or depressed	Thinking about the consequences/ outcomes of feeling depressed

episodes and fill in the diary immediately after you stop ruminating. This way, you'll capture what you truly think about when you are ruminating.

4. **Once you have completed the Brooding Diary, refer to it during your brooding session.** This will ensure that you are actually thinking about the important issues, and not something entirely different from your spontaneous, natural rumination. During your brooding session, force yourself to keep repeating the same thoughts over and over until you get sick of these phrases. Remember, there is no solution to rumination, so the best way to reduce its negative effect is to repeat it until it becomes stripped of meaning.

Intentional brooding works because you're taking back some degree of control over the brooding process. It's also a type of exposure, gradually making the ruminative thoughts less distressing and the process of rumination less anxiety-provoking. It helps you to objectify rumination—to treat the thoughts as "just thoughts" and not facts or truths about your life. As well, it's a way of experiencing the futility of rumination and its inability to lead to any kind of resolution; it is truly a "treadmill experience."

To make intentional brooding an effective mood repair strategy, note the use of the word *gradually* above. You will have to have a brooding session at least three to four times a week for a month to reduce spontaneous rumination and repair depressed mood.

This strategy has an extra benefit, in that you can use it to postpone brooding that tries to intrude on your day. When you find yourself starting to ruminate, write down the issue you were mulling over in your mind, and save it for your next scheduled brooding session. You can remind yourself: "I'll make note of that issue and really give it some time tonight during my brooding session. No need to spend time on it now; I may as well get back to my work. I've written it down and will really think it over tonight." This act of postponing your brooding until later is a good way to reduce the natural, spontaneous rumination that can significantly interfere in your daily work and relations with others.

Harold's experience of rumination on his depression and his perceived lack of faith can illustrate the use of the Brooding Diary and intentional brooding sessions. Harold began to spend 30 minutes daily trying to generate ruminative thinking like that depicted in his Brooding Diary (on the facing page). This "intentional brooding" was intended to allow Harold to postpone episodes of natural, spontaneous rumination until his more controlled, scheduled ruminative sessions. So one of the things he did was to think repeatedly, in a mechanical fashion, "What if I can't get to sleep? I'll feel more depressed." After he'd said that a few hundred times, the rumination began to feel like a "broken record" even to Harold, and he was ready to move on to some other aspect of rumination in his brooding session.

CAUTION If you feel more instead of less depressed after several attempts at using the Brooding Diary and scheduled brooding sessions, you should stop using this mood repair strategy. In this case, the sessions may be reinforcing negative, hopeless thinking that will only make you feel more depressed. The goal of Repair Strategy 26 is to strip rumination of its meaning, but if it is having the opposite effect on you, clearly it is not a strategy you should be using. Return to the other mood repair strategies in this chapter, and consider seeking professional help for your rumination (if you have not already done so).

Repair Strategy 27: Develop Your Distraction Skills

In the early years of research on rumination, distraction was considered the opposite of rumination. People who engaged in positive distraction activities when they fell into a depressed mood—activities such as doing something enjoyable, engaging in a hobby or some physical exercise, or making contact with friends—were thought to be responding adaptively to their negative mood state. Thus it was believed that distraction should reduce rumination, although the research findings have not always been so supportive.[1]

Brooding Diary: Harold

Thinking about causes for my sadness/situation	Thinking about how I am dealing with feeling sad or depressed	Thinking about the consequences/ outcomes of feeling depressed
It's my fault that I'm depressed. I shouldn't be depressed; nothing bad has happened in my life. I don't have a right to be depressed.	I feel so far from God; I can't feel His presence or blessing in my life.	God has abandoned me. I will never get into a right relationship with God; I'll never feel His blessing in my life again.
Depression is sinful; it's a sign of lack of faith. I'm depressed because I don't have enough faith in God.	I've lost all interest or motivation. I can't seem to pray or read my Bible.	I'll never get over this depression. I'll never regain purpose, motivation, energy, or enthusiasm for life.
God is punishing me for sin and unfaithfulness.	I have no purpose or meaning—no peace in my life.	People see me as pathetic—a weak and failed Christian.
Depression is a sign that I'm weak and sinful. I lack discipline or strength of character.	I can't sleep without sleeping pills. What if I get addicted to them? How can I function without being able to sleep naturally, as God intended?	I've committed the unforgivable sin of unfaithfulness; I am doomed to eternal punishment in hell.

Psychologist Susan Nolen-Hoeksema and colleagues have since refined the original view of distraction. They have argued that it may be critical to engage in one or two positive activities that truly absorb your attention, rather than to flit from one activity to the next.[1] In fact, there is experimental evidence that

> Distraction through absorption in an activity is the healthy alternative to brooding.

instructing people who feel sad to concentrate on thoughts or behaviors that are even neutral, but effective in diverting attention from negative thoughts and feelings, can reduce rumination and improve mood.[3] Thus the key to the success of distraction may be to become fully immersed in an activity, so that attention is directed away from rumination.

Use Repair Strategy 27 if . . .

- you have become much less active, spending a lot of time alone focused on feeling depressed.

- you have noticed even a slight improvement in mood when you are engaged in activities.

- you've found the behavioral mood repair strategies described in Chapter 5 helpful to some degree.

REPAIR STRATEGY 27 INSTRUCTIONS

1. **Think about activities that engage your attention and that require a moderate level of concentration and effort.** Driving, for example, is probably not ideal, because it is such an automatic behavioral sequence for most people that it siphons off only a small amount of attention. Something like strenuous aerobic exercise may be much more effective, because it captures more attention. But you would not want to choose exceedingly complex, demanding tasks, such as studying for a math exam, because any difficulties you have doing such a task could reinforce negative, self-critical thinking. When you are feeling depressed, a mentally taxing task may become overwhelming, and then you will start ruminating about failing the task (e.g., "Depression is going to ruin me, because I can't even concentrate on this simple math"). Thus moderately engaging activities are probably the best distracters for rumination. Take some time to discover the positive activities that are most effective in reducing or eliminating your bouts of rumination. Review the work you did in Chapter 5 to discover several behavioral strategies you could use as effective interventions for rumination.

TOOL FINDER   You may find doing some of the activities in your behavioral inventory (Repair Strategies 17 and 18) or focusing on boosting rewarding behavior (Repair Strategy 21) most helpful in dealing with rumination.

2. **Whenever you get into a ruminative cycle, get up and do something. Remember, you will gain nothing by sitting alone and ruminating.** The goal is to do something *right now* that cuts through the rumination and diverts your attention to another activity. This is the purpose of distraction: It's not to eliminate rumination permanently, but to serve as a strategy you can use at a particular moment to cease ruminating. Give it a try over a couple of weeks, and keep a record of your attempts. How effective was each activity you tried in capturing your attention and stopping the ruminative process "dead in its tracks"? Obviously, it will be a great idea to build up a repertoire of absorbing, highly effective distracting activities.

Getting Serious about Rumination

In the last several years, great strides have been made in understanding depressive rumination, its contribution to the persistence of depression, and ways to reduce its negative effects on people's lives. If you tend to be a ruminator when you are feeling low, practice using the rumination repair strategies described in this chapter. But be patient with yourself. Rumination can be a hard habit to break, since it is a well-learned mode of negative thinking for many people stuck in the blues.

TOOL FINDER Use the cognitive mood repair strategies in Chapter 4 to deal with specific negative thoughts and beliefs about rumination, and the behavioral mood repair strategies in Chapter 5 to help you use distraction and pleasant activities as alternatives to ruminating. The problem-solving approach (Repair Strategy 10) described in Chapter 3 can also be helpful for rumination, because it can help you find effective solutions to the life problems that may be a basis of your rumination.

> You can reduce depressive mood by turning rumination into reflection.

I should add one final note before leaving this topic: Some recent research indicates that *reflection* is the opposite of brooding. Reflection is a purposeful, inward focus on neutral or positive content—a process of cognitive problem solving directed at reducing depressive symptoms.[4] Reflection is a healthier self-focus that has been found to be related to a reduction in depressive feelings and symptoms. The next chapter presents acceptance and mindfulness meditation—mood repair strategies that encourage reflection rather than rumination.

7 capture the moment

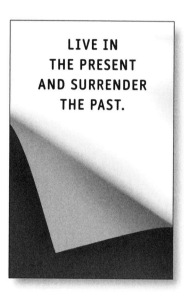

LIVE IN THE PRESENT AND SURRENDER THE PAST.

Whenever Charles felt depressed, he thought back to a job interview he'd had 5 years earlier with one of the largest and most prestigious information technology companies in the country. It was his dream job, the chance of a lifetime. He had made the short list from a long line of highly qualified applicants. The night before the interview, Charles could hardly sleep because of excitement mixed with anxiety. When he went in the next day, he felt a little groggy from lack of sleep. The interview was unusual in that applicants not only were asked the expected questions about their work experience and education, but were also required to solve some very complex mathematical and computer programming problems. Unfortunately, although Charles was a very bright and talented young man with a PhD in computer programming, he did not perform so well on these problems, and he was not offered a position with the company. Charles felt crushed, utterly defeated.

Even several years later, Charles often thought back to that interview and obsessed over his answers. He'd redo the problems in his head and wonder how he could have been so stupid not to see the answers. He'd dwell on his mistakes and conclude, "I just wasn't good enough or smart enough. I'm really not one of the best in my field; I'm just a mediocre programmer with no real talent. I was found out; finally my stupidity was discovered." Of course, Charles's rumination about this past failure and his inadequacies only deepened his depressed mood and drained away any confidence he had left in his abilities.

Tenshi also ruminated on the past during her periods of depression, but her rumination was of an entirely different nature. Tenshi was a highly conscientious, sensitive person who was very concerned not to offend other people. She would often go over conversations she had had with family or friends and worry that she might have said something rude or offensive. She would replay each conversation over and over in her mind, analyzing every word and the other person's reaction, trying to reassure herself that she had not said anything hurtful. This overthinking only made her feel guiltier, more depressed, and apprehensive about the future. But Tenshi's tendency to dwell on the past, what she had said and how she had acted toward others, was a ruminative tendency that had plagued her for years and drove her into long periods of depressed mood.

Until 2 years ago, Carla had thought she had the best marriage in the world. She'd just celebrated her 18th wedding anniversary with Jerry. But then he came home one day from work, tearful and visibly shaken. He confessed to her that he had had a one-night affair during a business trip several weeks ago. Since then he had felt tremendous guilt and regret, to the point where he had to confess and plead for forgiveness. Carla was shocked and devastated. Marriage fidelity was a high moral standard for her as a devout Catholic. The couple went for marriage counseling, and Carla and Jerry remained together, but the relationship was changed. Carla couldn't stop thinking about the incident. How could Jerry have betrayed her? What was the woman like? Was Jerry no longer sexually attracted to her? Was the other woman prettier? Would Jerry do it again? She thought about how it was all her fault for not being a good enough wife, asked herself how she could trust her husband, and wondered whether she could ever be happy again. Now, during her frequent bouts of depressed mood, Carla couldn't stop brooding over the affair, and yet she felt guilty for holding it against Jerry and worried about the future of their marriage.

Are You Dwelling on the Past?

Charles, Tenshi, and Carla had something in common during their periods of sad mood: All three suffered from ruminative thinking about some past failure or disappointment whenever they felt depressed. As discussed in Chapter 6, dwelling on the past in a very negative way is common during low moods. The mind of a person feeling down is highly selective, focusing on the negative and ignoring the positive. It's a biased way of thinking in which past losses, failures, regrets, and disappointments become magnified. Ruminators tend to think about the causes of a negative event, why it happened, what they did wrong, and the long-term adverse consequences. However, they are unable to think clearly about the past, because their depressed mood colors their perspective: Everything looks so much worse when we are stuck in the blues.

TOOL FINDER For more on why and how sad mood makes people focus on the negative and ignore the positive, see Chapters 1, 4, and 6.

Three problems are associated with this preoccupation with past losses and failures:

1. *Thinking about the past during a blue mood never resolves anything; it rarely leads to a solution or a settled feeling.* The past, of course, can't be changed, and the ability to think clearly is clouded by the negativity of depression. So the whole process becomes futile.

2. *If you think about past problems while you are down, the problems actually become magnified.* Because of the cognitive errors associated with depression (see Chapter 4), the consequences of the past will seem even larger and more significant here in the present and in the future. Carla, for example, became convinced that she would never get over Jerry's affair, and that it had changed their relationship forever.

3. *Dwelling on the past actually makes you feel more depressed.* As noted in Chapter 6, it's a false belief that you can "think through" some significant past negative experience and somehow come out feeling less depressed or having achieved some resolution of the past hurt. In fact, just the opposite will happen: The more you dwell on the past and ruminate about it, the worse you will feel.

> **Negative thinking about the past magnifies problems and fuels depression.**

Chapter 6 has presented a suite of rumination repair strategies that will also reduce any tendencies to dwell on past losses or failures. At the end of Chapter 6, I have mentioned *reflection* as a healthy way of thinking that counters rumination. An important feature of reflection is its focus on the present. Therapists and researchers have recently discovered that focusing on the present is a good way to head off ruminating over past negative experiences. A psychological treatment called *mindfulness therapy* has shown particular promise in helping people with depression become more reflective and focused on the present. Mark Williams, John Teasdale, Zindel Segal, and Jon Kabat-Zinn—the originators of this therapeutic approach, and the authors of a book titled *The Mindful Way through Depression: Freeing Yourself from Chronic Unhappiness*—define *mindfulness* as intentionally focusing attention on present moment experience in an accepting, nonjudgmental manner.

> **Mindfulness is focused attention on momentary experience.**

Through mindfulness training, you learn not to beat yourself up over past mistakes and failures, or to evaluate your negative thoughts and feelings in a catastrophizing, distressing manner. Instead, you learn to develop an accepting attitude toward all present thoughts and feelings that enter your conscious awareness. This letting go of evaluation and efforts to control your thoughts and feelings in the present moment interrupts the depressive ruminative cycle, leading to an eventual lowering of depressive mood. It is difficult to keep ruminating about past experiences at the same time that you are focusing on moment-to-moment thoughts and feelings in an accepting, nonjudgmental manner.

Mindfulness, then, is paying attention to the basic elements of our present experience—what we feel, think, or perceive at any given moment. It is allowing ourselves to become aware of an experience (even a negative or unwanted thought or feeling) as it actually occurs, rather than trying to control it or change it into what we want it to be. So we learn to stand back from our thoughts and feelings: We observe them and allow them to happen, but we do this in a noncritical, nonjudgmental manner, taking a welcoming orientation toward unwanted internal experiences.

Learning to distance yourself from the negative thoughts and feelings associated with the past, and to redirect attention to your moment-to-moment experiences—in other words, learning to live in the present rather than the past—has been shown to be an effective way to reduce the return of clinical depression in patients successfully treated with antidepressant medication.[1] These strategies appear to be especially helpful for individuals who experience occasional bursts of depressive symptoms during recovery. Furthermore, the effectiveness of mindfulness may be attributed to teaching individuals to take a more "decentered" observer's perspective toward their unwanted thoughts and feelings, and to be more accepting of their moment-by-moment experiences. So let's take a look at how you can use mindfulness to teach yourself how to live in the present, rather than fall into the rumination trap and dwell on the past.

> **Free yourself from negative thinking by being an observer of your thoughts.**

Use mindfulness mood repair if . . .

- you've had repeated occurrences of clinical depression, and you are currently in the recovery phase but still experiencing frequent depressed mood.

- you struggle with depressive rumination.

- you've had major losses, disappointments, or failures in the past, and you can't seem to let go of the experience.

- you have an interest in meditation and other contemplative exercises.

⤞⤞⤞ Repair Strategy ㉘: Cultivate Mindfulness by Heightening Awareness

As you are reading this page, what is happening to you? What are you consciously aware of at this moment? Are you fully paying attention to what you are reading, trying to grasp the concepts involved in mindfulness training? Or is your mind wandering to other things, like what to prepare for dinner or how much work you've got left to do? Maybe you're aware of feeling hungry or tired and thinking you need another cup of coffee. You could even be aware of how uncomfortable your seat is or whether you feel a pain in your arm. The fact is that at any given moment we all experience a host of thoughts, feelings, sensations, and perceptions, and yet we are aware of only a fraction of them. We cannot be consciously aware of the totality of our experience, and so our brains filter things out, selectively paying attention to one thing at any given moment and ignoring the rest.

When we feel depressed, we tend to filter out much of our present experience, because our minds are focused on some negative or disappointing experience in the past. When we are thinking about the past, much of our present, momentary experience goes unnoticed. Admittedly, we are aware of feeling depressed—but this becomes detached from the rest of our momentary experience, which gets filtered out and ignored because of our preoccupation with the past. What makes this process

> **A mind stuck in the past is insensitive to present experience.**

even worse is that our depressive thinking is highly biased for negative information, so that even our thinking of the past becomes a skewed misrepresentation of reality.

To counter this process, mindfulness therapy teaches people to pay attention to aspects of their current experience that they often ignore when feeling depressed. Instead of trying not to think negatively about the past—that is, trying to exert control over thoughts—mindfulness teaches individuals to let go of negative thinking, to cease

> **Wake up to the moment; be aware of your surroundings.**

trying to control it (e.g., "Let the negative thoughts float through your mind without effort"). This is done through attention-training exercises that focus on other, nonemotional aspects of momentary experience. This focus on other aspects of total experience leaves fewer attentional resources available for preoccupations with past events or for negative, critical self-reflection. In other words, learning to attend to more features of your momentary experience can deflect attention away from futile, maladaptive thinking that fuels depressed mood. Elevating your awareness of the present can thus become another effective mood repair strategy.

Think back to the last time you had dinner at one of your favorite restaurants—one where the food was exquisite, the wine list outstanding, the ambience soothing, and the service attentive. How mindful were you of this whole experience? Did you fully attend to each mouthful of food, savoring the taste and texture of the food? Were you able to stop and fully appreciate the smooth but full-bodied and slightly fruity flavor of the wine? Did you look around and appreciate how the design of the restaurant created a relaxing atmosphere? Can you actually remember what the waiter said and how you were treated? Or were you so engrossed in a heated conversation with your spouse, in thinking about a problem at work, or in worry about some family issue that you hardly noticed where you were, what you were eating, or how it tasted? Were you trapped inside your mind, rather than outside enjoying your experience? The fact is that there are two ways to experience a great restaurant, and the bill at the end doesn't change, however we've chosen to spend our time. Research on mindfulness has shown that we can be retrained to be more fully attentive to the present. And when we are being more aware of the present, we can't be thinking about the past. This is why soaking up the present, immersing your attention in the present, is an excellent mood repair strategy.

REPAIR STRATEGY 28 INSTRUCTIONS

Start learning mindfulness mood repair by practicing the art of appreciating the moment. The work of mindfulness therapists suggests five categories of mindful experience that you can use for your practice sessions. I suggest you begin with a specific activity that is unrelated to feeling depressed and is potentially pleasant, such as eating at your favorite restaurant.

Mindful Activity

1. **Make a reservation at your favorite restaurant, and then go with the intention of more fully appreciating the taste, smells, sounds, textures, and ambience of the food, wine, and décor.** Can you identify the different ingredients in the food by taste?

2. **Write a short summary of your restaurant experience, or even post a review of it online. Make note about how you felt while at the restaurant; you could even rate your level of happiness and sadness.** What did it feel like to be fully aware of your present, momentary restaurant experience? In *The Mindful Way through Depression,* Mark Williams and colleagues refer to this step as "paying atten-

tion on purpose, in the present moment, non-judgmentally, to things as they are"
(p. 54).

To cultivate mindfulness and learn to use this mood repair strategy effectively,
you have to be intentional and retrain your mind to become much more aware of your
surroundings.

Mindful Taste

1. Take a small piece of fruit, such as a raisin, a slice of apple, or a wedge of
   orange. First look at the piece of fruit in the palm of your hand, and really
   notice the different physical features of the fruit.

2. Then touch the fruit and note how it feels; smell it and see whether you can
   detect any aroma or fragrance.

3. Now place the fruit in your mouth and very slowly chew, paying attention to any
   taste sensations resulting from the fruit.

4. Then swallow the fruit, but be conscious of what you are doing and how it feels.

5. Sit back and think for a minute or two about this very simple experience. Appreciate your ability to taste food, as well as the experience of tasting it.

Mindful Breath

1. Set aside approximately 10 minutes, and find a quiet place where you will be
   alone and undistracted. Either sit or lie down.

2. Get comfortable, and begin by being aware of your body—the physical sensations in your back, arms, or legs caused by sitting or lying down on the floor.

3. After a couple of minutes, turn the focus of your attention to your breathing by
   noticing the rise and fall of your abdominal wall with each inhale and exhale
   of breath. Don't try to control your breathing;
   just let it happen naturally. Hold your attention to the action of your breathing. When
   your mind wanders, notice where it has gone,
   and then gently bring your attention back to
   your breath. This may happen several times
   during the 10-minute period, but that's OK; it's to be expected. Each time, bring
   your mind back to the breath in a noncritical manner.

> Intentional focus on the
> breath is critical training
> for living in the moment.

4. **Practice the mindful breathing several times a day. Each time, note how you feel during the exercise and immediately afterward.** With practice, are you finding the mindful breathing more helpful in shifting negative mood?

Mindful Pleasures and Beauty

In *The Mindful Way through Depression,* Williams and colleagues comment that "unawareness pervades our lives" (p. 60). That is, our minds often go on autopilot in everyday situations where overlearned ways of thinking prevail, leading to those old feelings of unhappiness and despair. There is likely to be much happening around you that is pleasant, positive, uplifting, and even beautiful—but you miss it, unmindfully, because you're stuck in the past. So this exercise involves consciously, intentionally making yourself mindful of the goodness that is happening around you. Examples could be the warmth of the sun, the beauty of a garden, the liveliness of a squirrel scurrying across your lawn, a kind or friendly comment by a stranger, and the smells of fresh air and spring; the list could go on indefinitely.

> Be mindful of the goodness and beauty around you.

1. **Several times during the day, ask yourself, "What pleasantness, goodness, or beauty am I missing that is happening at this moment, in this place?" Identify one or two positive features of the moment, and become fully aware of this thing of goodness. Focus on its effects on your senses (how it affects sight, sound, taste, touch, and smell).**

2. **Once you've fully experienced that stimulus, move on to another in a mindful manner, until you've spent 5–10 minutes cultivating mindfulness.**

As you become better at capturing the positive and pleasant in your momentary experience—better at stopping and "soaking in" kindness and goodness—you can use this as a mood repair strategy when feeling depressed. When Carla became aware of her negative preoccupation with Jerry's affair, she would shift her attention to what was happening at the moment and practice mindful attentiveness to positive or beautiful aspects of her current experience.

Mindful Routines

Yet another way to practice becoming more mindful is to attend deliberately to your current experience of certain routine, daily activities. Williams and colleagues give several examples, such as washing dishes, doing laundry, brushing your teeth, taking a shower, driving the car, and so forth.

1. **When you do these routine tasks, focus your attention fully on what you are doing, what it feels like, and how it is affecting you.** Rather than doing these activities in autopilot, be more fully aware of your actions.

2. **You could actually encourage your spouse/partner or another family member to be more aware of the mundane activities in his/her life. Then you could briefly discuss your various experiences of "the morning shower routine," for example.** Compare and contrast your different experiences of doing the same task. How have your experiences changed from day to day?

Obviously, these mindfulness exercises will not on their own repair a negative mood; paying attention to how you breathe or brush your teeth, for example, won't lift your spirits. But they will give you practice and training opportunities in being more aware of the present moment. And, together, they will introduce a powerful strategy to break the vicious cycle of rumination and negative thinking that fuels depressive mood. Developing an acute awareness of the moment shifts your mind from dwelling on past failures and disappointments to what you are doing right now, in this moment. Time shifting from past to present is a great way to avoid getting "stuck in the past."

> **Fill your mind with an awareness of your current actions.**

▸▸▸▸▸ Repair Strategy ㉙: Let Go of Negativity by Decentering

Cultivating mindfulness does not mean that you'll never have negative, depressing thoughts about the past. Negative thinking is a part of life; it's a natural feature of your emotional brain, and you can't erase your memory of past hurts, losses, or failures. So having negative thoughts is inevitable, but how you deal with them determines their effect on your mood state. *Decentering*, or taking the perspective of a nonjudgmental observer when you have such thoughts, is another key therapeutic strategy of mindfulness therapy.[2]

> **Negative thoughts are not truths, but instead interpretations of reality.**

One of the problems with depressive thinking is that we become engrossed in our negative thoughts, treating them as unquestionable facts about who we are and what we are worth. That is, we treat our negative thoughts as if they are truths rather than possibilities. When Charles felt depressed about his failed job interview, he experienced the thought "I have no talent or ability; I'm just not as intelligent as others in my field" as a truth about himself, an objective fact. Of course, this made the thought even more powerful in its effect on his mood state.

> **Don't criticize or blame yourself for having negative thoughts; accept them as fleeting events in your mind.**

One way to counter this all-consuming characteristic of depressive rumination is to develop a more impersonal, nonevaluative approach to your negative thoughts—that is, decentering. It is not easy to train yourself in decentering, but what you can do is try to catch your negative thoughts when you are feeling down or depressed.

Use Repair Strategy 29 when . . .

- you are flooded with negative, self-critical thoughts when feeling down.
- you tend to see your negative thoughts as truths—as accurate descriptions of yourself or your life circumstances.
- you are stuck in negativity and can't accept any other perspective.

REPAIR STRATEGY 29 INSTRUCTIONS

1. **Take just one of the negative thoughts that comes to mind when you're depressed, and talk to it in a "decentered" fashion. This involves learning to observe your thoughts and feelings as temporary, objective events of the mind, rather than as accurate reflections that are true descriptions of yourself.[2]**

   Tenshi, for example, was at work and feeling OK when she suddenly had this thought: "I wonder if I offended Jessica the other day by not commenting on her new tattoo. What if she is offended and doesn't want to hang out with me any more?" This bothered her, and she noticed herself becoming more anxious and distressed. Clearly, Tenshi was reacting to the thought "I wonder if I offended Jessica . . . " as if it were true—as if she did offend Jessica and her friend was upset with her. As well, Tenshi was taking this personally as an indication that she was an insensitive, uncaring individual. To take a decentered approach to the negative thoughts, Tenshi could say to herself,

> **Gently acknowledge negative thoughts as unwelcome guests that briefly occupy the center of your mind.**

   "Right now I am having an 'I offended others' thought. I often get these thoughts, and I've learned from past experience that they are untrue or don't really matter. They're examples of making mountains out of molehills. I'll just watch this thought float around in my head, like I would watch a leaf floating down a stream. I don't need to push the thought from my mind, because it's insignificant; I'll just passively watch it like I'm an outside observer."

Taking a passive, observing approach is one form of decentering, but another possible strategy is to decenter the negative thought with humor. This idea was inspired by psychologist Robert Leahy's approach to unwanted intrusive thoughts, as described in his book *Beat the Blues before They Beat You*. For example, Tenshi could talk back to her negative thought in the following way:

> "Oh, there's a 'maybe I offended a friend' thought again. Hi, old faithful thought. Welcome back into my conscious mind. You've been away for a few days. Can't say I really missed you, but I see you're back. How long would you like to stay in my mind this time? Feel free to stay as long as you want. Can I get you anything while you're hanging around—a cup of coffee, a snack? I'd love to stay and have a chat, but you know I have things to do. So I'm just going to get on with my daily activities, but feel free to make yourself comfortable. If you need anything, let me know."

Notice a few characteristics of this approach to repetitive negative thinking. First, the "I've offended someone" thought is treated as an object, an event of the mind, rather than reality. In the first scenario, Tenshi would simply acknowledge that she was having the thought, but would not get into whether or not the thought was true. She would refrain from trying to control, analyze, or suppress the thought of offending. She would simply allow the thought to be there in her mind, acknowledging that "a thought is a thought" and not a fact or truth, but a construction of the mind.

2. **Accept the thought in a nonjudgmental manner.** Tenshi wouldn't criticize herself for having the thought; she wouldn't try to control the thought or push it out of her mind. Rather, she would take a very accepting attitude toward the thought.

3. **Acknowledge the thought, but then get on with your daily activity.** In the second scenario (the humorous one), Tenshi would refuse to let the negative thought interrupt her, but would continue with her work whether or not she had the thought. Her assumption would be "If you want to stick around in my mind while I am busy with my activities, that's OK, because I can still get things done even if you decide to stay in my mind."

4. **Try to use humor.** In the second scenario, Tenshi would respond to the thought

as if it were another person. Humor can be a very effective strategy to remind yourself not to take your negative thoughts so seriously.

5. If your mind wanders back to the negative thought, reinstate decentering.

If you keep doing this over and over, you will become better and better at taking an impartial observer's perspective on negative thinking. When this happens, you will notice a positive effect on your depressive mood state.

➤➤➤ Repair Strategy ㉚: Express Your Negative Emotions

Mindfulness therapy also emphasizes the acceptance of negative feelings as well as negative thoughts. Although people are able to suppress negative emotions in the short term, this is not very effective in actually reducing the experience of sadness—and it may actually lead to more depressed mood over the long term, especially when a person stops exercising active emotion suppression. At the same time, another body of research shows that people with clinical depression experience reduced negative as well as positive emotion in laboratory settings when they use emotion suppression, although the positive emotion reduction is greater than the negative emotion reduction.[3] The implication of these findings is that the tendency for people to suppress their sad feelings may actually contribute to the persistence of sad mood, especially in people at risk for depression. Clearly, a more useful alternative is to teach people to express their negative emotions more fully during periods of low mood. Mindfulness therapy takes a step in this direction by emphasizing the importance of accepting spontaneous feelings—allowing them to happen, rather than trying to control these feelings or to suppress or avoid emotional experience.

> **Emotion suppression may contribute to greater depressed mood.**

More fully expressing happiness when you are happy and sadness when you are sad can be a helpful mood repair strategy, because it prevents the suppression or avoidance of emotion, which is known to contribute to negative mood. But what is recommended is *not* venting, or the exaggerated expression of emotion, or pretending to feel a certain way when you don't. Rather, it is allowing yourself to express a natural outflow of emotion in a genuine, authentic manner. So if you feel sad, allow the tears, the sad facial expression, or the pacing, if that is what feels natural. Expressive suppression, or actively inhibiting emotional expression, does little to prevent negative emotion. So fighting your tears, or trying not to look sad or depressed, could actually make you feel worse.

Use Repair Strategy 30 if you . . .

- have difficulty expressing your feelings.
- often fight back tears, trying hard not to appear sad and unhappy.
- pretend to feel fine when you're not.
- tell people you're OK when you're feeling terrible.

REPAIR STRATEGY 30 INSTRUCTIONS

1. **When you are feeling sad, accept that you feel sad. Don't try to fight it or control it, but let it take its natural course. If you feel like crying, have a good cry.**

2. **When you are done crying, get up and do something.** You may be in a social context where you can't freely express how you feel. In that case, steal away to the bathroom or some solitary place, have a good cry, and return to the social gathering when you are finished. Although this is not an ideal strategy, it's better than fighting back your emotions the whole evening.

In my clinical practice, I often have clients who become tearful during a therapy session. I always stop the session and encourage the clients to let themselves express their feelings. I don't continue with therapy, ignoring that they are on the verge of tears. I tell them that I'm not afraid of tears, that it's OK to express their feelings. Practically every time I've used this strategy, the client has cried for a few minutes, and then we seem to be able to get on with the session agenda. On the few occasions when clients have tried to fight back their emotions, a barrier seems to go up, and we make little progress. So learning to accept your spontaneous emotions, and to allow their natural expression, can be a very useful mood repair strategy. Ask yourself these questions: "Am I fighting back, pretending to feel something I don't feel, trying to hide my feelings from others? Or am I being true to myself, letting my momentary feelings take their natural course, expressing the way I feel in a genuine manner that is appropriate to my culture and the present social context?"

> Don't fight back the tears, but instead allow a free expression of genuine emotion.

▶▶▶▶ Repair Strategy ㉛: Find Peace and Solace through Meditation

In mindfulness therapy, meditative practices play a pivotal role in freeing an individual from the "gravitational pull" of depression by reminding the person that it's "okay to stop trying to solve the problem of feeling bad" (Williams et al., *The Mindful Way Through Depression*, p. 3). Based on the rich history of Buddhist meditation, mindfulness meditation seeks to raise awareness of the present moment through clear, deliberate, accepting, and nonjudgmental attention to a single object of experience. Williams and colleagues note that focusing on a single object of experience, rather than trying to deal with a multitude of competing demands, is an effective way of calming and steadying the brain. Individuals in mindfulness meditation are taught to focus their attention on the breath, the hands, or even the entire body (through a process called *body scan meditation*, discussed below) as the single object of immediate experience. Research has shown that mindfulness meditation has a positive calming effect on centers of the brain that deal with enhanced attention, as well as those that regulate positive and negative emotion. Although mindfulness is an effective treatment for anxiety and depression, whether meditation practice is critical to its effectiveness is unknown.

> **Mindfulness meditation can have a calming, positive influence on emotions.**

Many excellent self-help books provide advice on mindfulness meditation. A few suggestions are *The Mindful Way through Depression* by Mark Williams and colleagues, *Peaceful Mind* by John McQuaid and Paula Carmona, *Full Catastrophe Living* by Jon Kabat-Zinn, and *Buddha's Brain* by Rick Hanson. In explaining this type of meditation, Kabat-Zinn states that it is not a set of instructions to practice, but rather a process that involves your whole being. The foundation of mindfulness meditation is the adoption of a receptive attitude that is nonjudgmental, patient, open to new experience, trusting, nonstriving, accepting, and willing to let go. This last phrase means that you do not try to manipulate your experience, but instead "let [your] experience be what it is and practice observing it from moment to moment" (Kabat-Zinn, *Full Catastrophe Living*, p. 40). However, Kabat-Zinn also emphasizes the importance of exercising self-discipline and commitment to purposefully cultivating a receptive attitude toward mindfulness.

Use Repair Strategy 31 if you have . . .

- an interest in more contemplative exercises like yoga.
- a "racing mind"; that is, you're always thinking, worrying, or ruminating.
- difficulty relaxing, feeling calm, or being at peace.

REPAIR STRATEGY 31 INSTRUCTIONS

There are two aspects of mindfulness meditation. The first is a specific focus on the experience of breathing, and the second is a more general focus on bodily sensations.

Meditative Breathing

1. **If you have never meditated before, it is best to start out with a brief meditative session (about 5–10 minutes) once a day, and then gradually increase the time to about 30 minutes once a day.** Pick a time of day when you have the fewest demands on your time (early morning, later in the evening, lunchtime, etc.). Find a comfortable, quiet place to sit alone, where there are no distractions. Make sure that your clothing is not tight and uncomfortable; also, most people feel more relaxed with their shoes off. Dim lighting is preferable to the glare of fluorescent lights.

2. **You can sit in a chair or cross-legged on a cushion on the floor. Whatever you choose, your back should be straight and your chest open, so you can breathe easily and fully. Shift your body around until you feel a comfortable position— one in which you are centered over your lower body, and your head is raised gently upward so your eyes can focus straight in front of you.** Your body should be relaxed and firm, but not rigid and tense. If you notice any tension in a part of your body, let it go. Relax to the best of your ability. You can keep your eyes open or closed, although the latter is probably better at the beginning to help you concentrate.

3. **It is recommended that you begin meditation with a *focus on the breath*. Start by noticing how you are breathing, without trying to change it in any way.** Take your time and let yourself get into the present moment of the breath. Allow yourself to breathe in and out naturally, without rushing or controlling your breathing. Focus on the physical sensation of the breath in your belly. Notice how your belly rises as you breathe in and falls as you breathe out. Try to stay focused on the changing physical sensations in your abdomen for the full duration of each breath: inhaling, a pause, and then exhaling. If you have difficulty sustaining your attention on the abdomen, you can switch to the physical sensation of the breath in your nostrils. Notice the sensation of air coming in through your nose and then passing down your body to the abdomen. Do you notice anything about the breath, the temperature of the air, the feeling of inhaling and then exhaling?

4. **Your mind will wander, probably repeatedly, when you meditate. It may simply drift about aimlessly, or you may start to think or plan about the day's activities, or even some problem in your life.** Don't think of this as a mistake or failure, but accept it as a natural way in which the mind works. Gently notice what you are thinking about, and then softly redirect your attention back to the breath. Refocus on the rising and falling movement of your belly in response to each in-and-out cycle of breathing. Throughout your meditative experience, you want to cultivate

patience, kindness, and acceptance toward yourself, no matter how often your mind wanders.

5. **It is suggested that you repeatedly practice meditative breathing for a sustained period of time until you have worked up to 30 minutes or so daily.**

Once you are comfortable with mindful breathing, there are other meditative practices you can use to expand your repertoire. For example, you can use the mindful taste exercise discussed previously under Repair Strategy 28. In this case, the purpose is to use the focus on the fruit to create a relaxed, meditative state.

Body Scan Meditation

Developed by Jon Kabat-Zinn, body scan meditation is another exercise often taught in mindfulness therapy.

1. **Start again with a focus on the breath and the sensations it produces in the abdomen.** Your attention is focused on the rise and fall of the abdominal wall as breath enters the belly on the inhale and leaves on the exhale.

2. **Having connected with the physical sensations in the abdomen, now shift your attention to the physical sensations in the left leg, following them down to the left foot and toes.** Observe any sensation associated with specific parts of the left leg, such as the sense of contact, tingling, warmth, or even numbness felt in the hip, calf muscle, ankle, foot, and each toe. Be slow and patient, taking time with each part of the left leg. Now breathe in and, on the inhale, follow the breath as it moves through your body into your abdomen; then imagine it passing all the way through into your left leg, foot, and toes. Continue "breathing down into your toes" this way for a few minutes, and then, on the exhale, focus gently on the feeling in the bottom of your foot—possibly its contact with the floor. You continue with this shifting attention to the toes or ankle on the breath in, and then the bottom of the foot on the exhale.

3. **You can repeat this pattern as you shift attention to the right foot and other parts of your body—the pelvic area, the lower and upper back, chest, shoulders, arms, hands, and face.** When you become aware of tension in any part of the body, you can breathe in the sensation when you inhale, and then release it on the exhale.

4. **After you've scanned your whole body, spend a few minutes being aware of your breath moving freely in and out of your body.** Body scan meditation is frequently done lying down, so you might have the sensation of falling asleep.

▸▸▸▸ Repair Strategy ㉜: Consider a Place for Prayer

If you are a person of faith in which prayer plays an important role, you may be more comfortable with meditative prayer than with the Buddhist-inspired mindfulness meditation previously described. Not all prayer is the same, and depending on the type of prayer, it can have a positive or negative impact on emotional well-being. Four types of prayer have been identified: *ritual, petitionary, conversational,* and *meditative.* The first two types of prayer have been associated with increased rumination and negative emotion, whereas conversational and meditative prayer are associated with positive emotion and well-being. In a recent study of 177 British church attenders, frequency of meditative prayer was one of the few religious variables associated with self-reported positive mental health.[4] Thus there is some evidence that meditative prayer may be a positive coping strategy that has mood repair capabilities, although more empirical research is needed to establish this relationship. Meditative prayer is a more nonverbal, receptive type of prayer than the others; it is seen as an interchange with God rather than a personal monologue activity. It involves characteristics such as "feeling" God, thinking quietly about God, spending time worshiping God, reflecting on the Bible or other sacred texts, and listening to God for his answer to prayers. In meditative prayer, a person is not confessing sin, asking for forgiveness, expressing gratitude, or requesting guidance. The focus is on experiencing prayer, of having an experience of God.

Use Repair Strategy 32 when . . .

- religious faith plays an important role in your personal life and values.
- you already engage in prayer on a fairly regular basis.
- you engage in spiritual and religious practices (such as reading sacred scriptures; attending church, synagogue, or mosque; and the like) where prayer is emphasized.

REPAIR STRATEGY 32 INSTRUCTIONS

1. As with mindfulness meditation, it is often helpful to focus attention on a single object. In this case, it may be an image of an accepting God, some attribute of God, or a single verse or phrase from scripture.

2. Follow the steps for meditative breathing, with the exception that you focus on some attribute of God rather than on your breath. You might find it helpful to start your session by focusing on your breath and then shifting your attention to your chosen sacred attribute or image of God. It is better if you can hold your

attention to a single matter of faith, such as a verse or phrase of scripture, than if you switch back and forth between several spiritual objects of focus.

3. **Refrain from prayers of confession, contriteness, or repentance.** I recognize that confession and repentance are important in matters of faith, and they do have a place in the life of believers. However, for meditative prayer to have a positive mood repair effect, you need to maintain a positive, uplifting, praiseworthy orientation toward your prayer. Prayers of confession and forgiveness require a focus on personal mistakes, failures, and guilt. This will only intensify your attention to negative and self-critical thinking, which would make your depressive mood worse rather than better.

4. **The positive mood repair benefits of meditative prayer will become more evident when you engage in frequent, daily prayer.** The mood-lifting effects of meditative prayer are more likely to occur when it becomes a daily habit. Thus it is important that you choose a time and place in your day when you will not be distracted by other tasks and responsibilities.

The emotional benefits of prayer are still not understood scientifically. In the British study mentioned earlier, the frequency of prayer was not a significant predictor of positive mental health, but instead it was the type of prayer that was most important.[4] So what may be important is not how much you pray, but rather the quality of your prayer sessions—that is, whether you are able to achieve a state of meditative prayer.

Living in the Moment

When we are feeling depressed, we are often trapped in the past, ruminating about our failures, disappointments, losses, and mistakes. We can get caught in a perpetual cycle of self-criticism and negativity, leading to the experience of being stuck in the blues. This chapter has presented a number of strategies for averting rumination and depressed mood. Based on mindfulness therapy, these mood repair strategies involve a shift in attention from a futile reliving or rethinking of past losses and failures to a concentrated focus on the present. The key, as we have seen, is the adoption of a nonjudgmental acceptance—even heightened awareness—of immediate, momentary experience. This attentional shift from ruminating about the past to fully accepting and appreciating the experience of the moment can pull us out of the trap of negative thinking.

> **The mindful approach embraces a nonjudgmental openness to all life experience.**

To review, the first three strategies in this chapter—heightening momentary awareness (Repair Strategy 28), letting go of negative thoughts (Repair Strategy 29), and expressing/accepting negative emotions (Repair Strategy 30)—can all be employed for immediate repair. When you feel depressed, you can use these strategies "on the spot" to repair your mood. Repair Strategies 31 and 32, mindfulness meditation and meditative prayer, are longer-term practices that involve a change in lifestyle. By practicing either of these types of meditation, you will be enhancing emotional well-being more generally. The benefits on negative mood result from incorporating a time of meditation or prayer into your daily living.

Mindfulness, then, is a journey. It involves a change in your perspective on emotion and on life itself—from living in the past and trying to control the present, to concentrated awareness, acceptance, kindness, and patience toward your immediate physical experience.

8 ponder the past

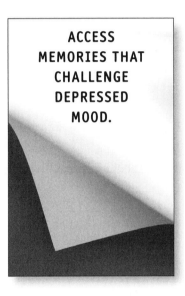

ACCESS MEMORIES THAT CHALLENGE DEPRESSED MOOD.

What do you tend to remember when you're feeling down or depressed? Most people struggling with low mood find it quite easy, if not entirely automatic, to think about past losses, failures, and disappointments, and almost impossible to remember their successes, accomplishments, and enjoyable times. There is a very close connection between the human memory retrieval system and emotions. When my colleagues and I want to induce feelings of sadness in our experiments on emotion, we often ask participants to think of a past loss or disappointment to get them into a negative mood state. Of course, the opposite approach is used to induce happiness or reduce sadness: We ask participants to think of a past accomplishment, success, or very enjoyable experience.

You will recall from Chapter 7 that Charles, Tenshi, and Carla all felt more depressed when they remembered past negative experiences. Charles remembered his failed job interview; Tenshi would rehash a possible mistake in almost every conversation with a friend; and Carla would think back to her husband's informing her of his one-night affair. In each case, negative memories triggered and/or intensified feelings of sadness. All three of them found it very helpful to learn to live more in the present. But sometimes even positive experiences from the past can become negative memories and exert a subtle but significant effect on mood. André, a college freshman, was very lonely and sad on many occasions during his first year away from home. He would think back to his friends and good times in high school, which you might think would be positive memories that should make him feel better. But they were actually negative memories, because he was remembering the loss of the good times: "Those great ol' days are over; I'll never be as happy again. I wish so bad I could turn the clock back. I was so happy back then, and now I'm so miserable."

At other times a negative memory can represent a difficult, even traumatic, loss or failure that determines current mood state in a clear and direct manner. Leah had spent the last 20 years struggling with frequent bouts of intense sadness. Eight years ago her oldest daughter, married and with two school-age children, had passed away after a year-long struggle with illness. Leah had devoted an entire year to looking after her daughter and her family through a long period of medical treatment. Then she was with her daughter during the last couple of months, when the prognosis for recovery was grim and her condition was terminal. Despite some healing with the passage of time, Leah still recalled that year vividly. Although she could remember some good times, her reminiscing was dominated by memories of loss, tears, and despair. Even 8 years later, a day didn't go by without Leah's having at least one crying spell over the loss of her daughter. She still had regular contact with her granddaughters, but each encounter brought back a flood of distressing memories.

Memory has a powerful effect on emotions, because the memory structures of the brain have strong neural links to emotion centers. This tight coupling of memory and emotion has been demonstrated not only in our mood induction research as described above, but in hundreds of laboratory studies in which people are more likely to remember negative memories when they are sad, and these memories in turn intensify a depressive mood state. However, research has also shown that people can use memories to change the way they feel. That is, you can feel less sad if you alter negative memories or improve access to positive memories. So the mood repair strategies in this chapter show how you can use your memory system as part of your mood repair toolkit.

Reminiscing about the Past

People who feel depressed or who are at higher risk for depression have a greater tendency to recall negative personal information and/or greater difficulty recalling positive personal information than others do. Interestingly, this applies not only to personal memories but also to impersonal information, such as a previously learned list of positive and negative words. In our research, we even found that typical university students who were made to feel sad for only a few minutes exhibited this bias toward recall of negative memories. Although the findings are a little less consistent on this, people may actually recall negative material more quickly when they are feeling depressed.

What all this means is there may be such a quick and automatic tendency to remember negative experiences from the past when we feel sad that we can suddenly find ourselves thinking about a negative experience without having tried to call up the memory.

A second characteristic of memory recall during low mood is called *overgeneralized memory*. In autobiographical memory experiments, individuals are presented with a list of cue words and are asked to recall a specific event associated with each cue word. The personal memory should be something that happened to them at a particular time and place, and that lasted a day or less. What has been found consistently is that people in a depressed mood tend to recall generalized or categorical memories, whereas those who aren't depressed recall specific memories of events involving particular times and places.[1] This finding is important, because remembering past events in an overgeneralized manner could have a negative impact on mood repair.

Let's say that research participants are presented the cue word *enjoy* and then asked to recall a personal memory associated with it. An example of a generalized memory might be "I always enjoy a good party," whereas a specific memory would be "I enjoyed John's party at the dorm last Saturday night."[1] The memory of John's party can lift mood more. This may happen partly because the specific memory contains more sensory-rich information, which can be reexperienced more vividly than a vague, generalized memory and thus can have a much greater emotional impact. Specific memories are also closely associated with other positive memories (e.g., John's party may remind you of other great parties or of people you met at parties who have become good friends) and so also lift your mood. Overgeneralized recall, in contrast, has been linked to poor problem solving and difficulty imagining future events, and it may be a marker for vulnerability to clinical depression.[1] Researchers have a lot more to learn about how the quality of a memory affects emotion regulation. Nevertheless, it would be prudent to assume that specific positive past memories have the best chance at improving a negative mood state.

> Positive specific memories may provide the best antidote to a depressive state that is fueled by overgeneralized negative memories.

Cognitive restructuring, through which you challenge thoughts that fuel depressed mood, can take advantage of the mood repair power of specific memories. The technique depends partly on learning to generate specific memories of past positive and negative experiences. Typically when people are feeling down, they generate overgeneralized statements such as "I always fail," and "Every time I try something new, it turns into a disaster." Cognitive therapists teach their clients to challenge these overgeneralized ideas by examining the specific details of past events. Trying to recall actual times, places, and specific events that represent "failing

> During low moods, negative memories tend to be vague and ill defined, and these qualities make recall of the past less accurate.

at something new" can correct a biased overgeneralized memory with more accurate, specific recall. André, when he thought about his last year in high school, tended to think in general terms about having a good time rather than actual specific events from his past. This generalized memory recall made his sadness and loneliness worse.

TOOL FINDER   Strategies based on cognitive restructuring are presented in Chapter 4.

A third feature of depressive memory is *difficulty with disengaging or inhibiting* the processing of negative material. In other words, when you are feeling down, you may have trouble letting go of negative memories and shifting your mind to something else. You may even have difficulty disengaging from irrelevant material, which would increase the tendency to have unwanted thoughts. This inability to inhibit negative and irrelevant information could lead to rumination and hinder your ability to use effective mood repair

> During a sad mood, you can get locked onto a negative memory and have difficulty letting go.

strategies to reduce negative emotion. Why is it so hard to let go of negative memories during a depressed mood? It's difficult mainly because the negativity of the memories matches the negativity of the mood state.

TOOL FINDER   Rumination, and mood repair strategies that target this form of negative repetitive thinking, are covered in Chapter 6.

Use the memory mood repair strategies presented in this chapter if you . . .

- get stuck in depressive rumination about past losses, failures, and disappointments.
- have significant regrets in your life.
- have difficulty thinking about positive memories when you are feeling down or depressed.
- feel stuck on particular past negative memories.
- have selective recall of your personal past.
- have mild, occasional periods of feeling blue.

▸▸▸➡ Repair Strategy ㉝: Retrieve Specific Positive Memories

When André reminisced about the good old days in high school, those memories triggered sadness, because they elicited related thoughts about missing all his old friends and how lonely he currently felt. But there is good reason not to give up on positive memory recall as a mood repair strategy for sadness, especially if you typically experience only mild to moderate bouts with the blues. The strategy described here will train you to retrieve specific, sensory-rich positive memories—the type that are more potent in countering depressed feelings.

REPAIR STRATEGY 33 INSTRUCTIONS

1. **Write down a list of 10 or more positive or happy personal past memories when you are in a positive (or at least neutral) mood state.** You could review the behavioral inventory of positive activities or your Hourly Behavior Record from Chapter 5 for examples of recent experiences that gave you a sense of accomplishment or enjoyment. You should have a mixture of past positive experiences that involved everyday experiences (such as an enjoyable conversation with a close friend last week, or praise from your boss about a project you completed) and positive major life events (such as a great Disney World family vacation several years ago, a complete recovery from surgery, or a big promotion). If you feel as if you're rarely in a positive mood, ask a close friend or family member to help you generate a positive memory list. The important point is to get this list down now, so you can use it when you *are* feeling depressed. If you don't, or if you generate the list while you are feeling blue, your recalled memories are likely to be weak and ineffective.

> Don't wait until you're feeling depressed to try to recall positive memories for the first time.

2. **It is important for each positive memory to be detailed, including specific information about the time, place, and circumstances in which the positive experience happened.** It is particularly critical to recall what you did to make the positive event happen and what positive consequences were associated with the experience.

   For example, Leah wrote, "I had a good visit from my surviving daughter last week." Unfortunately, this positive memory made her feel worse, because it reminded her of her other daughter (the one who had died). Instead, Leah needed to write something like this:

CAUTION If you struggle with frequent bouts of moderately severe depression, or if you have a history of clinical depression, don't try to recall happy memories to make yourself feel better. Positive memory recall may actually make you feel worse. Recalling happy memories can be an effective sad mood repair strategy, but only if you suffer *occasional, less intense* periods of sad mood. Positive memory recall may be ineffective for moderate to severely depressed individuals or may even make them feel more depressed for various reasons. Clinically depressed people may recall mainly overgeneralized or less vivid positive memories, which aren't very effective in repairing mood; they may start to ruminate if they are asked to look inward at all; or they may be reminded of how bad their current situation has become.[2] *Thus simply recalling past happy memories when you are feeling down may not make you feel better, and it could in fact make you feel worse.*

> **Trying to think of happy memories can actually make some people feel more depressed.**

"Last Wednesday afternoon, Joan (my younger daughter) came over, and we went shopping. I saw a dress that she tried on and really liked it, so I bought it for her as a gift. She was so happy; we chatted about some more things and all the funny things my grandchildren are doing. We went to my favorite café and had a delicious cappuccino. I felt so happy that my daughter and her family are living close by and that we get along so well. It was a warm, sunny spring day, and this made the whole experience even better. I noticed we seemed to be practically the only mother–daughter couple in the mall having such a good time."

There is evidence that if you can get enough detail so you can actually imagine the past happy memory (i.e., if you can actually visualize it rather than think about it in words), it will be an even more potent mood repair strategy.[3]

3. **Keep the list of positive memories in a small notebook that you can carry with you, or load it into your smartphone.** When you notice a slump in your mood, take out the list and select a positive memory to think about. There is no formula for which memory to choose. It should be a memory that captures your attention at the moment, and that you can recall in sufficient detail to cause a shift in your mood state. Using the same positive memory over and over, or recalling it in a general way, will weaken the memory's influence on your mood. Also, focus on the memory as intently as you can for at least 5–10 minutes. If you can get yourself into the memory, it won't take long for you to feel a shift in your negative mood.

4. **Each time you use positive memory recollection to repair a sad mood, pay close attention to the meaning you bring to the memory. Think about what role you played in making this positive experience happen, and focus on how you actually felt during the experience.** For Leah, it was important to think about what she had done to create such a close relationship with her younger daughter, and how she was now enjoying this relationship in her senior years. It is also critical to remind yourself that you'll have more positive experiences in the future, just like the happy memory you are thinking about right now, as well as other enjoyable or successful experiences you've had in the past. You can remind yourself that there is nothing in life that is so catastrophic that it will permanently wipe out any chance of even occasional moments of enjoyment or success. Even in the direst of human circumstances, almost everyone is able to escape into some pleasant experience, even if only briefly and temporarily. Remembering your past successes and other pleasurable experiences can be a reminder that your life is not one continuous state of despair, but that it has been—and will continue to be—punctuated with moments of happiness.

> Happy experiences rarely happen completely out of the blue; we all play some role, however minor, in our personal experiences. So consider the role you have played in creating positive memories.

You will need to practice positive memory retrieval frequently before it will be effective in repairing sad mood. Also, you'll need a variety of happy memories to use at different times; obviously, you'll quickly get bored and lose interest if you use the same happy memory every time you engage in mood repair. As well, negative thinking will sometimes intrude into your mind, distracting you from the positive memory. When this happens, acknowledge the negative thoughts, and then gently redirect your attention to the happy memory—possibly focusing on its meaning and implications for you both now and in the future. Writing down some further details about the happy event may help you concentrate on it more fully. However, you can probably only hold on to a positive memory for 5–10 minutes before you lose concentration. But that should be enough time for the positive memory recall to have some positive effect in reducing the intensity of your sad mood state.

CAUTION Positive memory retrieval should be used along with other mood repair strategies, to bolster their effectiveness. It is not the most potent mood repair strategy in your toolkit, and it will not be particularly effective if used alone.

⫸ Repair Strategy **34**: Realign Your Negative Memories

As mentioned in earlier chapters, negative memories can seem like vultures waiting to swoop down on you when mood is low. Their tendency to enter the mind may be somewhat unavoidable, but there are better ways to think about the negative past that reduce its impact on depressed mood. That's what this strategy is all about.

Although the effects of negative memory suppression are far from settled, it is probably safe to conclude that trying not to think about a past negative experience is a maladaptive mood repair effort (see the sidebar "The Dangers of Memory Suppression" below). Memory suppression is particularly adverse for those who experience frequent bouts of low mood, are prone to negative emotion, or are clinically depressed. You might find that you will actually think about these things less if you cease your memory suppression efforts. So the

> Don't suppress your negative memories; rather, gently acknowledge their presence.

best advice to everyone is, don't try to suppress negative personal memories but instead *to harness the negativity of unpleasant memories by working with them in a more productive manner.* The current mood repair strategy focuses on improving your recall and evaluation of past negative memories, because clearer, more accurate mem-

the dangers of memory suppression

If you have some painful memories from the past, it is understandable that you would try not to think about them. However, active attempts not to think about a negative memory may actually be counterproductive: They may make the memory even more powerful and easier to remember. *In fact, trying not to think about a negative memory, or to suppress the memory, may increase your access to negative memories more generally.* A British study discovered that individuals who had depressive symptoms and were told to suppress a single negative childhood memory actually recalled other negative personal memories better than depressed individuals who did not suppress a negative childhood memory.[4] The depressed individuals who suppressed the memory also subsequently experienced more negative intrusive thoughts about the memory than the depressed individuals who did not suppress it. Other research studies have found that nondepressed individuals can suppress negative personal memories quite effectively, at least for a few minutes, but that adverse long-term effects may be associated with repeated suppression.

ories for past experiences—even the hurtful ones—will reduce their negative effect on your mood. This strategy is also designed to counter any tendencies to suppress negative memories, which we know has maladaptive effects on the blues (see the sidebar on the facing page).

Use Repair Strategy 34 if you . . .

- experience frequent unwanted intrusive thoughts about past negative, hurtful, and/or distressing experiences.

- try not to think about certain experiences from the past, but they keep coming back into your mind.

- have negative or painful past experiences, or regrets about experiences, that make you feel more depressed when you remember them.

- have a poor or vague memory of a past experience that you nonetheless find distressing.

REPAIR STRATEGY 34 INSTRUCTIONS

1. **When you spontaneously begin to think about a past negative experience, acknowledge that the memory has entered your stream of consciousness. Recognize the memory for what it is: It is *thinking about* the past but not *reliving* the past, because what's past is behind you.** It is important that you label this current experience for what it is: "I am having thoughts about a particular past experience." It is also important to remind yourself that memory is always selective; it is never perfectly accurate. For all of us, memories are reconstructions of the past. If you don't believe me, try this experiment: Pick a common family experience from the past, and then ask your family members what they remember. You will find that no two people recall the incident in exactly the same way.

2. **Now prepare to harness the negative memory by creating a Memory Reconstruction Form like the one shown in part on the next page (or print one out from *www.guilford.com/clark7-forms*).**

3. **Start filling in the form by using the left column to list all the things you remember clearly about the event.** What happened, when, and under what circumstances? Who was involved in the incident, and what did they do? What caused the event to take place? What was your role in causing the negative experience? What impact did the experience have on you? No doubt you will find this column relatively easy to complete, but it is probably the first time you've written out a

Memory Reconstruction Form

Things I remember clearly about the negative experience	Things I've forgotten about the negative experience
1.	1.
2.	2.

narrative of the event, so you may find that you remember new facts about the experience as you write down what happened.

4. **Now stand back, take a look at what you've written, and ask yourself these questions:**

"How am I being selective in what I remember about this experience? Am I exaggerating the importance of some things and minimizing other aspects of the experience? Am I blaming myself too much for causing the negative experience or at least not preventing it from happening? Am I overly focused on the negative impact, or am I not thinking clearly about its long-term consequences?"

5. **After you've evaluated what you've written in the left column, reexamine the memory and try to search for aspects of the past experience you may have forgotten. Write these in the right column.** This will be much more difficult, because now you are trying to recall aspects of the experience you may not have thought about in years. If others were present at the time of the incident, or you remember talking to them about it at the time, ask them what they remember about this event. It may be they can remember aspects of the experience you've long forgotten. No doubt the list of "forgotten" material will be much shorter than the list in the "remembered" column, but that's fine; recalling even a couple of new features may help you arrive at a more balanced recollection of the past.

6. **Ask yourself these questions:**

"What changed as a result of this experience? Was there anything positive

that came out of this experience? Did I learn anything, or was there a positive change in me because of this experience? Was anything worse prevented
because of this negative experience? Overall, how much better or worse am I
today because of this negative incident in the past?"

7. **Now you're ready to arrive at a new understanding—what we call a *reappraisal*
of the past—based on what you've written in the two columns.** This part of the
exercise focuses on developing a new construction, a new way to think about the
past experience. Ask yourself these questions:

   "What's the most realistic, balanced way to remember this past experience?
   What are the present-day consequences, both positive and negative, associated with the event? What would be the most helpful way for me to remember this experience?"

On the same sheet of paper where you recorded your initial, negative memory
or in the spaces below, write down your new, more balanced reconstruction of the
memory:

a. Old, selective memory of the past event:

_____

_____

_____

b. New, more realistic memory of the past event:

_____

_____

_____

8. **Now it's important to remind yourself of this new reconstruction of the past
whenever you feel depressed and the negative memory intrudes into your
thinking.** When you are thinking of this past experience, gently focus on your new
memory or way of recalling the past experience—the new aspects of the memory
you've discovered as a result of the memory reconstruction method. Spend a few
minutes thinking about the past incident in this new way, possibly even adding to
or elaborating on your new memory. Then turn your attention to some new task
or activity. Give yourself permission to divert your attention to the task at hand by

acknowledging, "I've spent enough time with the memory today. I'll come back to it tomorrow or at some future date. It will always be there for me to observe and remember." Note the mood repair impact of this new approach to remembering the past. Are you better able to let go of the loss, hurt, and disappointment of the past and refocus on the present?

Ruth was in her early 60s and looking forward to retirement. Financially secure, active, and fully engaged in life, Ruth felt devastated when she was diagnosed with Stage II breast cancer. She underwent a lumpectomy, followed by a course of radiation and chemotherapy. Her oncologist declared the treatment highly successful and said Ruth could expect to live a long and satisfying life. Her annual checkups for the next 3 years reaffirmed that she was free of cancer. However, Ruth noticed that she now experienced many more periods of depressed mood, when all she could think about was her experience of being diagnosed with cancer. What Ruth discovered when working on her negative memories of this experience was that she tended to remember (1) the repeated mammograms that kept coming back positive; (2) the shock of being told by her oncologist that she had breast cancer; (3) the terrible fatigue and nausea of chemotherapy; (4) her fears that it would recur and her life would now be shortened; (5) all the women she met who had had recurrences; and (6) women who had died of breast cancer.

Ruth struggled at first to remember forgotten aspects of her cancer experience. Eventually, however, she was able to write down (1) the names of all the women she had met who had more than 10 years of productive lives after treatment for Stage II, or even Stage III, cancer; (2) an account of the positive prognosis she received from the oncologist; (3) a list of the medical sources indicating that her type of cancer had some of the highest survival rates; (4) the positive personal changes resulting from her experience with cancer, such as a fuller appreciation of life, more compassion toward others, a closer relationship with her husband and family, and a deeper spiritual life; and (5) a greater resolve to fulfill her aspirations and life wishes now, rather than waiting for some future retirement date.

Ruth realized that her old memory of her cancer experience had led her to think, "It's so unfair that I should be stricken with cancer. I'm sure to die soon and miss so many opportunities, like seeing my grandchildren grow up and enjoying the freedom of retirement with my husband." However, her new recollection of her cancer experience led to the following conclusion:

"I can treat this cancer as an early warning, because I know people who live their life well after cancer. None of us have a guarantee of tomorrow, which could involve some unexpected calamity or even death. What my cancer has taught me is to enrich my connections with loved ones and to get the most from each day. Without cancer, I might have continued to live my remaining years in a fog—wasting my days on things that don't matter, always thinking I have lots of time for the important things in life."

Ruth continued to relive her cancer experience, especially during periods of low mood. But now she could use her new, more balanced memories to reinterpret the experience in a more realistic, healthy manner. Since negative memory recall played a key role in Ruth's depressed moods, achieving more balanced and realistic memories was an effective mood repair strategy for her.

Navigating the Past

We all have both positive and negative experiences in our past. When we are feeling low, there is a strong tendency to remember the losses, mistakes, and disappointments and to forget or minimize the pleasures and successes of the past. It is also natural during low periods for memories of past losses and failures to flood our minds, exacerbating our depressed mood state. Efforts to deal with this overwhelming negativity, such as forcing ourselves to think happy thoughts or suppressing the memories, may actually make matters worse. This chapter has presented two mood repair strategies that you can use to make remembering the past a more helpful way to lift yourself out of the blues. You will, however, need to use other mood repair strategies in dealing with negative and painful past experiences that contribute to feeling depressed.

TOOL FINDER If your past negative experience is causing actual problems in your present life, you will need to review the problem-solving strategies in Chapter 3. You may be experiencing a lot of negative thoughts and beliefs about yourself because you are dwelling on the past, and so you'll need to do some more cognitive mood repair with the strategies in Chapter 4. Depressive rumination often occurs when people have significant negative memories; consult Chapters 6 and 7 if you get stuck in remembering. Finally, the strategies in Chapter 13 will be useful if you engage in extensive avoidance because of what has happened to you in the past.

9 embrace your dreams

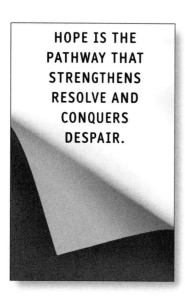

HOPE IS THE PATHWAY THAT STRENGTHENS RESOLVE AND CONQUERS DESPAIR.

Have you ever worked hard at something—given it all you had—and you still didn't succeed? Maybe during your student days, despite long hours of study on a difficult course, you couldn't manage a grade better than a mere pass. Or you've been trying to diet, but the pounds aren't coming off. Or you've tried everything to get yourself out of financial debt, but each month you're going further into the hole. Maybe you've had a recurrence of a serious medical illness, or you have a child headed in the wrong direction despite your best efforts and advice. We have all faced these types of circumstances when failure seems to stalk us at every corner, and when this happens, the natural tendency is to lose hope—to feel discouraged, helpless, and depressed. During such times, there is a strong urge to give up, "throw in the towel," and lose heart or abandon our commitment to our goals and aspirations. The loss of hope has been described as an inner death leading to a sense of meaninglessness and despair.

Marianna knew what it was like to lose hope. A 38-year-old woman with a bachelor's degree in business, in good health, and married with no children, Marianna had worked for the past 15 years at a midlevel job in her city's commerce department. It had been her first job after college, but in the last 7 years she'd been feeling very dissatisfied with it. The job had started to feel tedious and unrewarding, and so she started working extra hard—taking on more projects, working late and on weekends, jumping in to give coworkers a hand, and taking courses toward an MBA—all in an effort to get a promotion or find a new employer. And yet, in the last 5 years, Marianna had been overlooked for every promotion and had not been offered any job she'd applied for. For whatever reason, her intelligence, enthusiasm, strong work ethic, and good organizational skills had not been recognized, and she now felt trapped in a dead-end job—possibly for life. Marianna was losing hope and was now just going through the motions at work. Her dreams of completing her MBA and becoming a financial consultant had faded, and Marianna was noticing that her times of depressed mood were getting longer and more frequent.

Loss of hope is common in clinical depression. But it can also be a part of everyday sadness, and when hopelessness is unaddressed it can lead to persistent despair. Fortunately, we know a lot about what makes people feel hopeless: negative expectations for the future, lack of commitment to goals, and low assessments of their own ability to achieve and reach goals. The mood repair strategies presented in this chapter target these critical elements to turn hopelessness into hopefulness.

Hope: A Wellspring of the Soul

From ancient times, the world's great wisdom literature has been filled with references to hope as an essential element of the human spirit. For example, the Bible speaks a lot about hope; one example is the verse "We have this hope as an anchor for the soul, firm and secure" (Hebrews 6:19a, New International Version). More recently, science has turned its attention to the nature of hope, especially its role in emotional states like depression. Aaron T. Beck, the founder of cognitive therapy (see Chapter 4), was also one of the first psychiatrists to systematically research the role of hopelessness in clinical depression and suicide risk. He considered hopelessness—the belief that there is no point to living, that there is nothing to look forward to, and that one will never be happy—to be a core element in suicidal thinking. Numerous studies have since found that hopelessness is a specific characteristic of depression, and it has even been proposed as a defining feature of some types of clinical depression.

C. R. Snyder at the University of Kansas has offered the most detailed explanation of hope to date.[1] He defines *hope* as a positive motivational state derived from three beliefs people have about themselves: (1) that they can successfully achieve positive life goals and avoid negative life outcomes; (2) that they have a plan for how to achieve these objectives; and (3) that they are capable of using this plan to reach desired outcomes. Snyder argues that hope is a personality characteristic, with high-hope individuals having more positive and active feelings about engaging in a variety of future goal pursuits. Thus high-hope individuals feel greater friendliness, happiness, and confidence. Low-hope individuals, on the other hand, have more negative feelings as well as more apprehension and passivity about the pursuit of future goals (i.e., a greater sense of helplessness). Low-hope individuals also have a more negative expectancy about the future and believe they are less able to achieve desirable or prevent undesirable outcomes. According to Snyder, negative emotions are the products of unsuccessful goal pursuits, whereas positive emotions are the results of successful goal pursuits. In his review, Snyder notes that high-hope individuals fare better in academics, athletics, physical health, psychological adjustment, and psychotherapy than low-hope individuals do. He also notes that increasing hope has been shown to raise positive emotions and to lower negative emotions.

The *pursuit of goals* is a fundamental characteristic of human nature that plays a critical role in determining our level of hope. All human actions are goal-directed; the desire to attain positive goals or aspirations reinforces some behaviors, whereas the desire to prevent negative outcomes influences others (such as avoidant behavior). Think for a moment of the importance of goals in your life. Your goals might be to have more friends, a better job, greater intimacy in your marriage, more leisure time, better physical health, longer life, closer relations with your children, greater financial security, or the like. All of us have literally dozens if not hundreds of goals, ranging from the very specific ("I want to reduce salt intake in my diet") to the more abstract or generalized ("I want to have a closer relationship with my children"). Goals can also be immediate ("I want to do well on tomorrow's exam") or long-term ("I want to be financially secure in retirement"). Whether short- or long-term, specific or general, goals influence our behavior and directly affect our emotions. And when we fail to attain important goals or come to believe we can't achieve our goals, loss of hope and depressed mood are most likely to occur.

> Hope requires investment in specific highly valued life goals and aspirations.

There are various ways in which goal attainment can go wrong and lead to depression. Selecting a very lofty goal with a low probability of success is more likely to lead to disappointment than setting a more moderate but attainable goal is. For instance, wanting to be president of the company when you are a clerk's assistant is more likely to result in disappointment than aspiring to be the office supervisor. Also, defining your goal in vague, abstract terms ("I want to have a successful career") is less likely to be effective than adopting goals that are more concrete and specific ("I hope to be promoted to assistant manager within the next 2 years").

Failure to adopt any meaningful life goals can also be a problem. A significant loss, such as death of a spouse, divorce, or job loss, can threaten cherished goals and leave you feeling that life has no meaning. This in turn can make you feel hopeless, as if there is nothing more to live for.

A second characteristic of high hope is *commitment to a plan of action*. A plan of action involves thinking about how to act now so you can reach your goals in the future.[1] You need to know what to do to reach your goals, and it's likely that the more pathways to success you can envision, the better. At the same time, losing your way and not being able to think through a course of action for goal attainment will lead to a sense of helplessness and eventually hopelessness. Marianna, for example, believed she had run out of options. She had taken various steps to improve her chances of promotion, but nothing had worked out. She didn't know what else to do; she had no "Plan B." When people are stumped and have no plan of action, they usually give up. A sense of helplessness sets in, followed closely by hopelessness. This entire state can become a self-fulfilling prophecy: You believe nothing will work out, and you give up, so of course your goals are not achieved. In this way hopelessness ends up creating the very conditions you were wanting to avoid. That is, you end up being stuck and going nowhere, because you have given up doing anything to get yourself out of the situation.

A third characteristic of high hope is a *belief that you have the capacity to pursue a course of action and reach the desired goal or outcome.*[1] This belief is also known to psychologists as *self-efficacy*. Self-talk such as "I can do this," "I know what to do," or "If I just keep working at this, I know I can succeed," is evident in people who are hopeful about achieving a goal. High-hope people have confidence in themselves and can visualize themselves reaching their goals. When barriers or difficulties arise, they persevere because they believe they will succeed eventually. Not surprisingly, low-hope people have little confidence in their ability, and their self-talk is characterized by thoughts like "I don't know what I am doing," "I'll never succeed," or "I just don't have the talent or ability to succeed at this." Their lack of belief in themselves means that they quickly give up when faced with even the smallest adversity or setback.

The mood repair strategies in this chapter focus on building hope for the future as an antidote to the emptiness, discouragement, and helplessness that often prevail during periods of loss, sadness, and despair. High hope can reduce depressive mood by countering these negative beliefs and expectancies, which play such an important role in keeping people stuck in the blues.

Use the hope-building strategies in this chapter when you . . .

- are pessimistic about your future.
- view your future as empty or bleak.
- feel helpless and/or have given up on trying to improve your life circumstances.
- have no life goals or ambitions.
- feel there is no meaning or purpose to your life.

▸▸▸▸ Repair Strategy ㉟: Confront the Crystal Ball

You can begin rebuilding a sense of hope right now, by taking stock of your level of hope for the future. It involves looking into your personal "crystal ball" and examining your desires for the future.

REPAIR STRATEGY 35 INSTRUCTIONS

1. **Think of some of the things in your life that you've lost hope of achieving.** Are there positive, desirable outcomes or goals that you once wished to pursue, but now believe you can't achieve? What are they? How important or valuable are these goals for you? Are there negative outcomes or circumstances that you now think you can't avoid?

2. **Ask yourself whether there are any positive goals you remain hopeful about attaining in the future.** Are there hopeful things happening in your life, no matter how small or insignificant? Have you been able to avoid some negative outcomes that have worried you? Is there anything about the future that gives you reason to hope, that is associated with a positive expectancy?

3. **Guided by the previous questions, make a list of the negative expectancies, outcomes, or goals in your life that seem hopeless to you, and list the life expectancies, outcomes, and goals that remain hopeful.** You can create a form like the partial Crystal Ball Inventory shown below, or print out a complete form from *www.guilford.com/clark7-forms*.

   If you've been feeling depressed for a while, you might find the right ("hopeful") column of the Crystal Ball Inventory much more difficult to complete. Try completing the "hopeless" column when you are feeling depressed, and the "hopeful" column when you are in a more positive mood state. Use brainstorming to generate as many "hopeless" and "hopeful" examples as you can. As with past experiences, you could ask your spouse/partner, a close friend, or a family member to help you generate your list—someone who knows something about your life goals and aspirations.

Crystal Ball Inventory

How the future looks hopeless to me	How the future looks hopeful to me
1.	1.
2.	2.

TOOL FINDER   Brainstorming is explained in Chapter 3 (Repair Strategy 10).

4. Now place an asterisk beside the entries that are really important to you—the goals associated with high personal value. Ask yourself the following questions:

"Am I exaggerating the level of hopelessness in my life?"

"Have I overlooked or discounted the hopeful things in my life—the things that are going right and are likely to work out fine?"

"Do I have a greater chance of achieving some important life goals than I have been expecting?"

"How can I be more realistically hopeful about some of the things on my 'hopeless' list? Have I really exhausted all possibilities?"

"Are there some goals that I hoped to achieve that should be radically changed or even eliminated?"

It would be helpful if you wrote down your responses to the preceding questions.

5. To use your Crystal Ball Inventory for mood repair, read over the inventory and your evaluation whenever you feel down or depressed. Focus on whether there is more hope in your life than you are feeling at this moment. Add to the list any new "hopeless" thoughts that are preventing you from thinking about your positive goals, or new "hopeful" thoughts that indicate you are making some progress in your life. You will need to use some of the other mood strategies in this chapter to boost the repair capability of the crystal ball exercise.

Marianna's Crystal Ball Inventory is shown on page 150. As can be seen from Marianna's lists, much of the hopelessness in her life centered on her disappointing work experiences. Career achievement was important to her, and she clearly felt defeated in reaching her goals of advancement, meaningful work, recognized success, and fulfillment in this area. Because her career was so important to Marianna, she focused almost exclusively on it, and so she felt that her entire situation was hopeless and depressing. And yet it is clear that Marianna had a lot of other life goals where progress was evident. A focus on the right column indicates that Marianna was living in more hopeful circumstances than she had realized.

The point of this exercise is not to deny the negative things—the disappointments that engender a sense of hopelessness. Rather, the objective is to arrive at a more realistic, balanced perspective in which you can truly recognize the positive

Crystal Ball Inventory: Marianna

How the future looks hopeless to me	How the future looks hopeful to me
1. <u>Career advance</u>: Having a management career in the financial service industry.	1. <u>Education</u>: I'll complete my MBA with honors.
2. <u>Retirement</u>: Building a secure retirement fund.	2. <u>Physical appearance</u>: I've succeeded in improving and maintaining my physical fitness and appearance.
3. <u>Meaning</u>: Making a difference in this world through my work and career.	3. <u>Marriage</u>: My marriage is secure and continuing to grow in depth and intimacy.
4. <u>Success</u>: Having career success that is recognized by my family and friends.	4. <u>Social relations</u>: I continue to make friends, and my girlfriends continue to plan winter trips with me.
5. <u>Fulfilling work</u>: Feeling challenged and excited by my work.	5. <u>Personal finance</u>: Our financial situation continues to improve year after year.
	6. <u>Recreation and leisure</u>: I have a busy social and recreational calendar; over the years, there seems to be more and more to do on the evenings and weekends.
	7. <u>Charity</u>: I started volunteering to teach remedial math to teens at risk for dropping out of high school.

parts of your life. If you can do this, you will feel less hopeless and consequently less depressed about yourself and your current situation.

⟫⟫⟫➡ Repair Strategy 36: Define Your Life Goals and Values

When was the last time you really thought about what is important in your life—what you really value? How would you like to be remembered by others? What do you want to succeed or accomplish in this life? What activities do you find most meaningful? What brings you the greatest amount of happiness or life satisfaction? In studies of daily mood, researchers have found that people spend the greatest amount of time doing things they least enjoy (e.g., work, commuting), and much less time doing the things that bring the greatest amount of happiness (e.g., socializing, relaxing, sex).[2] Can you relate to these findings? Do you spend more time on things that are least enjoyable or even least important to you, and less time on the things that really matter in your life? This question relates to your personal values and aspirations in life. If it helps you explore your personal values, you could imagine your funeral and what you would like people to say about you and your legacy. On the other hand, are there negative aspects of your behavior—certain habits or ways of relating to others—that you don't want as your legacy or don't want others to remember?

Hope requires that we have life goals and aspirations, and these, in turn, are derived from our personal values—that is, from what we consider meaningful and worthwhile. Our values can center on a variety of domains, such as family, social relations, wealth, health, popularity, spiritual depth, and charity. So the questions now are these: What are your values, and how focused are you on their attainment?

> **Personal values guide goal selection, which gives meaning and purpose to life.**

Norman, a single man approaching 30 years old, felt lost and aimless, suffering frequent bouts of depressed mood and despair. He had tried to enroll in college several times, but on each attempt he would quickly lose interest and drop out after a few weeks. He had spent most of his 20s partying and drifting from one recreation-oriented job to another (ski instructor in the winter, tennis pro in the summer). Between jobs he would return home and live with his parents, spending most of his days playing video games and his evenings drinking with friends. But Norman found that he was becoming more and more isolated as his friends got jobs and settled down to raise families. He was forced to hang out with a younger crowd who saw him as the "old man." The problem for Norman was that he had no meaningful life goals. He wanted to go back to college, but kept changing his major because he had no career aspirations. The only things in his life that brought enjoyment were partying, video games, and volunteer work at the tennis club. Norman had not discovered his personal values and so was going through life without long-term meaningful goals. No wonder he felt down and depressed much of the time: He was not only stuck in the blues, but stuck in a time bubble more appropriate for a teenager than a young adult.

You may not find this exercise necessary if you already have a good sense of your personal values. Perhaps you already know what is important to you, but the problem may be that you feel blocked and frustrated in your attempts to achieve life goals and lead a fulfilling life.

Use Repair Strategy 36 if . . .

- you feel that you're drifting through life.

- you're not sure what is important or what you really want out of life.

- you once were goal-directed, but you're not sure any more.

- you struggle with motivation.

REPAIR STRATEGY 36 INSTRUCTIONS

1. **To begin work on your life goals, start by defining your personal values that guide goal selection.** You can use the Defining Values Form below to help you with this exercise, or print out the form from *www.guilford.com/clark7-forms*. You can also review some of the self-monitoring forms you completed in Chapters 2, 3, and 5, to identify positive and negative activities to list in the upper half of the form.

    We can take Marianna's situation as an illustration of a values assessment. In the top left quadrant of the Defining Values Form, Marianna included going to the gym, doing well on a graduate exam, dining out with her husband, and having coffee with friends as positive, life-satisfying activities. Activities she placed in the top right quadrant as associated with dissatisfaction included working late at night alone in the office, being pressured with more work by her supervisor, eating junk food meals because of time constraints, and being stuck in traffic.

    After considerable thought, Marianna wanted to be remembered as a highly successful and productive professional who had achieved far more than was ever

Defining Values Form

	Positive/pursue	Negative/avoid
Activities that affect life satisfaction		
How I could be remembered		

expected; who could accomplish a great deal with calm and efficiency; who was understanding and considerate of others; and who could relax, laugh, and enjoy life. She wrote these down in the bottom left quadrant of the Defining Values Form. At the same time, Marianna realized there were several things she did not

> **Goal setting begins with taking inventory of your personal values.**

want as part of her legacy, such as being remembered as a frustrated and angry person, a lonely workaholic, a person always stressed out and overloaded, a person completely self-absorbed and insistent on her own way, or a stingy and miserly individual. These things went into the bottom right quadrant of the form.

As Marianna evaluated her Defining Values Form, a number of life values became apparent to her:

- The importance of a challenging and productive career
- The ability to work calmly and efficiently
- Opportunities to share good times with a few close friends
- A deep and abiding relationship with her spouse
- The ability to relax and enjoy leisure time
- The desire to avoid frustration, stress, and the feeling of being unable to cope

2. **Once you've established a list of meaningful life values, you can construct more specific goals based on these values.** It is important to set goals that are specific and consistent with your values. A goal can be challenging, but it must be doable, and you must know what has to be done to reach that goal. That is, you must have the skills, ability, and opportunity to pursue the goal actively. For example, having a goal of running a 4-minute mile is not realistic for me, given my age and physical limitations. However, it does make sense to have a goal of running 10 km under 1 hour, given my running history. A larger, long-term goal can also be broken down into subgoals that can be attained in a shorter period of time.

Marianna, for example, wanted to relax more and enjoy her leisure time. Given that she was currently working almost every evening, she set a goal of taking at least two evenings a week to focus on relaxation and leisure. She could use the problem-solving approach described in Chapter 3 (Repair Strategy 10) to construct a plan for dealing with her workload so she could free up two evenings a week for relaxation. She could then implement her plan, evaluate its success, and determine how well she was fulfilling her desire to enjoy more relaxation and leisure in her life.

➤➤➤➤ Repair Strategy ㊲: Construct a Positive Imagery Script

Building hope to counter depressed mood requires an ability to recognize what is hopeful in your life, a willingness to question generalized feelings of hopelessness (Repair Strategy 35), and a commitment to pursue specific, realistic goals based on cherished personal values (Repair Strategy 36). These strategies can be enhanced by actually visualizing a hopeful future, rather than just thinking about your goals, dreams, and aspirations. *Mental imagery* refers to the experience of "seeing with the mind's eye" some past or future event.[3] Because it is sensory-based, it differs in detail and quality from simply thinking about an event. Imagery is also much closer to dreaming and could be thought of as "daydreaming." Let's say you really want the job you were just interviewed for. Using mental imagery would involve picturing yourself actually working in an office at this company, sitting at your desk, and starting the first day of work, rather than just thinking about getting the job in a more detached, intellectual fashion.

Recently researchers have discovered that mental imagery has a much more powerful impact on emotions than simply thinking in words does: It acts as an emotional amplifier. In other words, positive feelings are felt more strongly when positive future events are mentally visualized, compared to simply thinking about them.[3] Clinical researchers have also shown that positive imagery can reduce depressed mood.

> **Imagery is a mood amplifier; hopeful daydreaming can increase positive mood and reduce negative feelings.**

One way to develop a mental image and boost the mood repair capabilities of positive goal setting is a process called *imagery scripting*. This technique involves writing a narrative, a script, of what you see and feel in the imagined experience. The imagery script must be written from your perspective as the main actor, and it should be as specific and detailed as possible.

Imagery scripting is an essential strategy for building hope, and so it should be used if you've worked on any of the mood repair strategies presented in this chapter. It is hard to be hopeful if you can't imagine attaining your goals and aspirations.

> **If you are trying to build more hope, then positive imagery scripting should be a critical part of your mood repair strategy.**

REPAIR STRATEGY 37 INSTRUCTIONS

1. **Select a positive goal that is based on an important personal value. Write a narrative describing what you imagine it would be like to attain that positive goal**

in the future. Use the following suggestions to guide construction of your positive imagery script:

- How did you achieve the goal?

- Describe the situation or circumstances of the goal attainment. Who's present, where did it happen, and when did it happen?

- How did you feel about reaching the goal? Describe the positive feelings— the happiness, joy, and so on—you experience from achieving the goal.

- What are the positive effects resulting from the goal achievement?

- Include any ideas of what you'll do next. Where could this positive goal lead you?

Marianna could use positive imagery scripting to boost the mood repair effectiveness of her "increased relaxation and enjoyment" goal. The following would be an example of her positive imagery script:

It's Wednesday evening, and I've just finished cleaning up after dinner. Jim and I are sitting in the living room, and there is nothing planned for this evening. It's a little chilly, and so he turns on the gas fireplace. I change into my pajamas, pour a glass of wine, and curl up on the sofa wrapped in a comfortable blanket. I am feeling tired but contented after a busy day at work. I stare at the fire and feel the warmth of the heat on my body. I take a sip of the wine and enjoy its full-bodied flavor. The room is dimly lit, and I focus on the quietness of the room and the faint ticking of a distant clock. My body feels limp and relaxed after an enjoyable meal, a glass of good wine, and the warmth of the fire. After several minutes of soaking up the ambience and the realization that I can sit here for the next 2 hours, I pick up my novel and become engrossed in the story. Time slips away as I become thoroughly involved in this intriguing tale of love and mystery.

2. **After you construct a positive imagery script, it is important actually to use it as a mood repair strategy.** At times when you feel depressed, discouraged, or hopeless about your life, take the positive imagery script and spend a few minutes daydreaming about your goal.

3. **Take concrete action in working toward your imagined goal.** Positive imagery must be followed by actual behavioral change; that is, you must engage in actual work toward your goals. Building hope and overcoming the blues can-

> Dare to be a "dreamer" with regular positive imagery experiences that bring hope for the future.

not be achieved by simply daydreaming about a better future. You must also see yourself engaged in activities on a day-to-day basis that contribute to eventual goal attainment. For example, if your positive imagery script is having a close, fun, and memorable experience with your family, just daydreaming about a great family vacation won't be enough to make you feel better. You will need to do what it takes to make this dream a reality, such as to start saving, planning, and talking to family members about taking an exotic vacation together.

An example of using positive imagery as an actual mood repair strategy would be Marianna's taking a few minutes at work when she was feeling particularly stressed to imagine a time of relaxation by the fire. Just a few minutes of truly focused positive imagery can be enough to have a helpful impact on your mood. This can be done several times a day with different goals, so that the imagery doesn't become monotonous and stale. The other advantage of this type of daydreaming is that it will encourage hope and strengthen your resolve to work toward the positive goal.

➤➤➤ Repair Strategy ㊳: Engage in Mental Contrasting

A mild sad mood can actually have a positive impact on problem solving and goal attainment, if your expectations of success are high and you engage in a cognitive strategy called *mental contrasting*.[4] This process involves intentionally imagining a positive future goal, and then reflecting on obstacles or problems in the present reality that interfere with achieving the future goal. For example, a single woman imagines falling in love but then realizes she hasn't had a date in months, or a single man imagines increasing his social activities but has just moved to a new city and realizes that he has a very limited social network. Research has shown that when people feel sad but engage in mental contrasting, they have higher expectations for success and feel more energized in their commitment toward the future positive goal.[4] However, it is important to get the order correct: First imagine your goal or aspiration, and *then*

> Mental contrasting is an essential part of building hope, and so it should always be used when you are doing any of the mood repair strategies presented in this chapter.

think about the obstacles preventing goal achievement. *Reverse contrasting* occurs when a person dwells on the negative reality before thinking about the positive future, and thus has lower success expectancy and goal commitment. Reverse contrasting may be more likely to occur when a sad mood is more intense or when a person has low hope. Completing the previous hope-building exercises (Repair

Strategies 35–37) will help you avoid reverse contrasting, because they force you to work on goals and aspirations before getting into the obstacles to goal attainment.

Mental contrasting is a good example of a mood repair strategy that involves harnessing sad mood. It seems to work best when people are in a more reflective mode of thinking, as they may be during a sad mood. You need to be in the frame of mind where you can take time and ponder the challenges and obstacles to goal attainment.

REPAIR STRATEGY 38 INSTRUCTIONS

1. **Go back to the work you did in Repair Strategies 35 and 36, and select a couple of positive future goals that are important to you.** If you didn't complete these earlier strategies, you'll get more out of mental contrasting if you go back and work on these other mood repair tasks first. Then elaborate on your positive goals, providing enough detail that you can clearly imagine what it would be like to achieve the goals.

2. **Next, think about two or three obstacles or difficulties in the present real world that would interfere with attaining one of your goals.** Again, elaborate on these obstacles, but think about what you can do to overcome the obstacles and attain the positive goal. Think about the goal in light of the obstacles and challenges; that is, mentally contrast them. Can you see yourself overcoming the barriers and being successful at attaining the positive life goal?

One of Marianna's life values was to have a closer, more intimate relationship with her husband. A specific goal related to this value was to plan at least one enjoyable activity together each weekend. This could be going to the movies, having dinner out, socializing with another couple, or something similar. Mental contrasting involved thinking about doing these activities with her husband, and then reflecting on real-life obstacles that would interfere in the pursuit of these experiences. These could include impending work deadlines that made her feel she should be working instead of being with her husband; feeling too tired to go out in the evening; her husband's reluctance to go out because he had other things to do; or limited money to spend on entertainment. It would be important for Marianna to engage in problem solving and come up with ways to deal with these difficulties that would enable her to attain her goal of sharing an enjoyable activity each weekend with her husband.

TOOL FINDER   For problem solving, see Chapter 3, Repair Strategy 10.

A Reconsideration of Hope

A loss of hope or positive expectancy for the future will deepen a depressed state and prevent recovery from it. High hope involves an investment in valued future life goals, a commitment to a plan of action for achieving these goals, and a belief in your ability to reach the desired outcome. This chapter has offered several mood repair strategies involving goal commitment that can boost hopefulness and reverse a depressed mood or sense of despair. However, being hopeful does not simply mean dreaming about a better tomorrow. It does involve action—committed work aimed at achieving a more positive future. Also, high hope does not mean that any of us will always get what we want. Sometimes our desires cannot be met, and at these times we have to learn to accept reality. Acceptance of that which we cannot change is another important part of living a hopeful life.

In addition, hope building does not occur in isolation from the mood repair strategies discussed in previous chapters. The following list suggests some ways you can combine other strategies with hope building to lift yourself more effectively out of the blues.

TOOL FINDER

- Use the cognitive mood repair strategies in Chapter 4 to deal with the negative, self-critical thoughts and beliefs that often accompany hopelessness.
- Use the behavioral mood repair strategies in Chapter 5 to take action so you can make real progress in fulfilling your dreams.
- Use the problem-solving approach in Chapter 3 to work through any obstacles associated with goal attainment.
- If you are avoiding difficult situations that need to be resolved before you can feel hopeful, see Chapter 13 on overcoming procrastination and other forms of avoidance.
- If you feel stuck in your hopelessness, you may be falling into depressive rumination. If so, consult the mood repair strategies in Chapter 6.
- And use the mindfulness strategies in Chapter 7 when you need to reach a desirable level of acceptance of things you cannot change.

Individuals with high hope do not spend their entire time focused on the future. Rather, it is important to achieve a perspective in which you also appreciate what exists in the present and can embrace acceptance. To achieve fulfillment and life satisfaction, each of us needs to work out for ourselves an optimal balance between being driven by our dreams with fortitude and determination to overcome the obstacles and setbacks that hinder goal attainment on the one hand, and acceptance, contentment, and appreciation of the present moment on the other.

> **Emotional well-being is a combination of hope for a promising tomorrow with acceptance of that which we cannot change.**

Finally, it is important to recognize that hope cannot be easily quantified or measured. It should not depend entirely on achieving a particular goal or desired outcome, which may or may not come true. Rather, the most important type of hope is a generalized expectancy of a meaningful, satisfying future life that will involve some positive goal attainment, as well as occasional disappointments that we can accept without hindrance to our quality of life. Hope, then, carries us along life's journey. Don Williams, Jr., an American novelist and poet, reminds us that "the road of life twists and turns and no two directions are ever the same; yet our lessons come from the journey, not the destination."

10 make connections

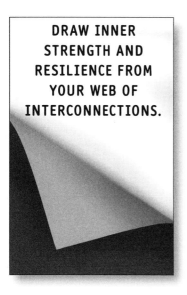

DRAW INNER STRENGTH AND RESILIENCE FROM YOUR WEB OF INTERCONNECTIONS.

Suzanne felt all alone. A year ago, she had reluctantly decided to retire after 35 years of teaching elementary school. Seven years earlier, she had downsized, moving into a townhouse after her husband suddenly passed away. She saw her two adult children only occasionally, because they had busy lives in distant cities. Suzanne had a couple of close friends from work, was active in her synagogue, volunteered for various community events, and had a sister and several relatives living in the same city. She was quite active most days, but Sundays had been the worst since Bill died. That was the one day when she spent more time alone and would feel the most depressed.

Since her retirement, Suzanne was experiencing even more times of feeling blue, alone, isolated from the world, and forgotten. Whenever she had social contact with a friend or was busy volunteering, she felt fine. It was the times she spent alone in her house, especially the afternoons, when she felt most lonely and depressed. Everyone around her seemed so busy, so engaged in their lives, so connected with each other in their work—and there she was on the outside, alone and left to fend for herself. During these times of loneliness, Suzanne felt particularly blue and found that she withdrew even further into her shell, cutting herself off from friends and family. She had a sense that this was the wrong thing to do, because it might only be making her more depressed; however, she had no interest in seeing others, no energy to pretend all was well, and no capacity to lie that she was enjoying retirement. When depressed, Suzanne believed that connecting with others was just not worth it—that she put more into relationships than she ever received in return. Suzanne was becoming more and more disconnected from the world around her, and it was taking a heavy toll on her emotional well-being.

This chapter focuses on social relationships and their effects on your mood state.

Psychologist Stephen Ilardi states in his book *The Depression Cure* that dependence on others is an innate, biologically based instinct that has been evident in all human societies from the beginning of time. Evolutionary psychologists contend that the drive to form social groups, such as families, tribes, communities, and countries, is a universal motive critical to our survival as a species. If you stop to think about it, we seem to enjoy ourselves most when we are around others—visiting friends, going to parties, dances, having dinner together, and the like. As humans, we are most resilient when we face hardships together, and most vulnerable when we are alone and isolated. The ability of individuals to survive the most horrific conditions imaginable, such as the extermination camps in Nazi Germany, can be credited in part to the tight-knit social connections formed between prisoners. And for centuries, jailers have known that solitary confinement is one of the worst punishments they can inflict.

> **The need for social contact is a universal human motive that is critical to survival.**

The mood repair strategies presented in this chapter are designed to help you reverse the automatic social withdrawal and avoidance response you may experience when you are feeling lonely and depressed. As the "Depression Makes Us Lonely" sidebar on the next page explains, doing nothing and staying at home alone will be the easiest choices when you are feeling blue. It takes considerable determination to break out of this habit. This chapter's mood repair strategies can help you break free of loneliness.

Use these strategies for working on social relationships if . . .

- social withdrawal, isolation, and avoidance occur when you feel depressed.
- you often feel lonely.
- you are often in conflict with friends, family, or colleagues.
- you feel awkward or uncomfortable around others.
- you lack confidence in social settings.

A Social Barrier Checklist

Check off the factors below that might be keeping you isolated. Knowing which of this "dirty dozen" of relationship busters is plaguing you will help you choose the best mood repair strategies for you.

❑ **Introverted personality:** *Have you always been a shy person who has difficulty connecting with others? Does social interaction come less naturally to you than to others,*

depression makes us lonely

Given the importance of social relationships to the survival of human beings, a condition like depression, which has such an adverse effect on social relations, might seem as if it should have become extinct long ago. However, depression may have survived in the human species because it does have at least one useful function: It causes us to conserve energy, and this may be connected to the neurophysiology of depression. When feeling depressed, we are motivated to withdraw and avoid contact with others, possibly in an effort to conserve energy and focus on feeling better. Stephen Ilardi has speculated that possibly this conservation function occurs because the brain mistakenly treats depression like an infectious disease. But the problem is that our immune systems are not under attack, and we don't need to conserve energy. Thus social withdrawal only amplifies the depression, making it worse rather than better. Psychologists Jeremy Pettit and Thomas Joiner, in their book *The Interpersonal Solution to Depression,* summarize research findings showing that the social relationships of people who are depressed are more negative and dysfunctional—characterized by more conflict, more arguments, more feelings of rejection, and less support—than the relationships of nondepressed people. Depressed individuals may be more impaired in their social skills (e.g., more passive and unassertive), and so less effective in their dealings with others. As a result, they may actually endure more negative reactions from others, as well as a withdrawal of their social support. So there may be some truth to a depressed person's belief that "nobody wants to associate with me when I'm depressed," but the reasons reside within the depressed person's negative interpersonal behavior. It's the depression, not the person, driving any rejection by others.

So science gives us some clues as to why it is so hard to force yourself to connect with others when you're feeling depressed. On the one hand, you are experiencing a natural urge to conserve energy by doing the thing that is easiest and less taxing. Staying at home alone is definitely the easiest. On the other, depression changes the way you behave socially, so that your interactions with others may not go as well as when you are feeling more positive. Thus the desire to withdraw is a natural consequence of feeling depressed.

requiring you to work at it—to be much more intentional in making connections with others? People who suffer from frequent and persistent depressed moods are often introverts. Although you can't change your basic personality (introversion has a strong genetic basis), you can use the strategies below to improve your social life and make more meaningful connections with others.

❑ **Social anxiety:** *Do you feel anxious or on edge when you are in social situations? Are there certain social settings that make you anxious, or do you feel generally uncomfortable in most interpersonal situations? Is anxiety holding you back from a better social life?* Most of us feel nervous or anxious around other people from time to time, but some people almost always feel anxious in social situations. If you are socially anxious, you probably feel highly self-conscious around others and are concerned that people are forming a negative opinion of you (e.g., that you are stupid, incompetent, weird, or unfriendly). These feelings can become so overpowering that outright avoidance of social situations or escape into solitude brings with it a sense of relief, safety, and comfort. You can use the strategies in this chapter to break out of your comfort zone and become more engaged with others.

❑ **Negative beliefs:** *Do you hold any negative beliefs about contacting your friends and family that are holding you back from making connections? Are you being overly negative about the importance of social contact in your life, or your ability to relate to others?* Do any of the following beliefs sound familiar to you?

- "I'm just not a people person."

- "It's too hard to meet people."

- "I'm a loner—the type of person who doesn't need relationships."

- "It's better, less stressful when I'm alone."

- "People don't want to be around me when I'm depressed."

- "Making contact with friends or family won't make me feel any better."

- "I'm such a boring person; nobody wants to associate with me."

- "My friends don't really like me; they just tolerate me."

> People who feel depressed believe that their social abilities are worse than they really are, whereas nondepressed people tend to overestimate their social skills.

- "It takes too much effort to socialize."

- "People can't be trusted; they'll just hurt you in the end."

TOOL FINDER   If negative beliefs like these are holding you back from being more sociable, you should revisit the cognitive mood repair strategies in Chapter 4. You will find the social mood repair strategies discussed below more effective when used in combination with the cognitive strategies.

❏ **Social devaluation:** *Have you lost your desire to invest in others? Have relationships become empty and worthless in your life? Have work, material goods, and career aspirations squeezed out your investment in creating a deep, multilayered social network?* Having multiple levels of closeness—from intimate family relations to more casual neighborhood or work connection—is a good protection against depression. However, our society tends to put greater value on things like earning more money and owning bigger homes or more luxurious cars than on relationships, even though relationships are stronger contributors to happiness than material possessions or career success. People stuck in the blues may find this imbalance worse, because it can push them to the point of not really caring about others or about whether they have meaningful social relations. When this happens, these people have entered the dangerous waters of social isolation and intense loneliness, where in turn they will feel depression even more intensely.

TOOL FINDER   Review some of the work you have done with the strategies for life goals and values in Chapter 9. These strategies can be used along with the social mood repair strategies presented in this chapter.

❏ **Excessive negativity:** *When you feel down, are you driving people away with excessive negativity? Do people see you as a complainer or a highly critical person? Do you always see the dark side to conversational topics?* As noted in Chapter 4, thinking tends to become negative during depressed moods. People who are depressed talk more negatively in their social interactions than nondepressed individuals: They often focus on more negative topics, or make more disparaging and belittling comments about themselves or other people. Not surprisingly, other people find this negativity distressing and may start to avoid the depressed persons, who then typically adopt the negative belief that others just don't like them. This has the predictable effect of worsening the depression and creating a vicious cycle.

TOOL FINDER   If this social barrier is relevant for you, you may need to make some changes in your social behavior by using the strategies in Chapter 5, along with the social mood repair strategies discussed below.

❑ **Fear of getting hurt:** *Are you avoiding others for fear of getting hurt? Do you have a tendency to take things too personally, and thus to feel hurt by other people more than you should?* People who are feeling low tend to become more sensitive to other people's remarks, which may stem from their negative self-view. Depressed individuals already feel bad about themselves, so they may be quick to interpret negative remarks from others as personally relevant and consistent with their negative self-view. *Or do you think you might be drawn to negative or critical people during your depressed moods?* Sometimes depressed people actually seek out negative feedback from others, which only prevents mood repair by increasing their depressive symptoms. If this is true for you, wouldn't it be better to associate with more positive, uplifting friends and family members?

❑ **People pleasing:** *Are you trying too hard to please your friends and family? Is this having an unwanted negative effect on the quality of your personal relationships with others?* Trying to please others can intensify depression. Basing your self-worth on the degree of love, approval, and acceptance you receive from others is a no-win situation, since it's difficult to know when people are pleased with you. Even at best, the approval and acceptance of others can be fleeting. Once you start trying to win friendship through "people pleasing," you have to keep doing it over and over again to deal with your uncertainties about where you stand with others. In the end you can become too submissive, even subservient; this may only cause others to devalue their relationships with you, or to take you for granted.

❑ **Fearing others' negative evaluation:** *Are you overly concerned about people's impression of you? Do you tend to assume that others think negatively about you? Do you avoid people for fear of giving a negative impression?* As noted previously, fear that other people will think badly of us is a core feature of social anxiety, but it also fuels avoidance of social interaction more generally. If you're convinced your friends don't really like you or don't want to associate with you because you believe they find you boring or unfriendly, you'll avoid them. But we can never know what people truly think of us, because none of us can read minds. So we all have to live with the unknowable—that is, with not knowing what people are truly thinking about us at any given moment. You may keep all your thoughts and opinions to yourself, because you do not want to hurt other persons or to give them a bad opinion of you. If you are gripped with fear of negative evaluation, you can use the social mood repair strategies to learn contentment in not knowing what others think.

❑ **Excessive reassurance seeking:** *Are you a "comfort seeker"? Do you demand reassurance that you are liked, loved, and valued? Do you think that this insistent seeking of reassurance and comfort may be driving others from you, and thus making you feel worse rather than better?* There are two ways in which the need for reassurance fuels depression: It is never really satisfying, so that persons with this need feel compelled to seek reassurance repeatedly, and it is often irritating to others. Researchers have found that frequent reassurance seeking is associated with more intense depressive symptoms, especially when it is combined with interpersonal stress (e.g., conflicts with a spouse or arguments with close friends).[1]

> **TOOL FINDER** You may find it necessary to use the strategies in Chapters 4 and 11, along with your work on social relations in this chapter, to overcome the habit of reassurance seeking.

❑ **The blame game:** *When you are feeling down, do you act differently toward others? Have you been waiting for others to change, rather than taking the initiative yourself?* There's no way to win the blame game, because we have limited control over other people's behavior. We can't force people to like us; we can show kindness and understanding toward others, but that doesn't ensure that they will like us. And we can't change people against their will. So blaming others doesn't really solve interpersonal problems or social isolation. It is simply shifting responsibility for the relationship onto the other persons, and then sitting back helplessly and waiting for them to change their behavior. As you know, you can wait a very long time for people to change; indeed, it may never happen. The alternative is to look inward—to ask yourself how you can use mood repair strategies to improve a relationship. This often means taking the initiative with your friends and family.

❑ **Self-initiated pressure:** *Are you able to be yourself in social situations? Or are you putting excessive pressure on yourself to play a different social role that is not natural for you?* We can't all be the life of every party. Nor can shy persons, for example, live up to the self-imposed expectation that they need to take the initiative in conversations, to talk about interesting things, and to ensure there are no silent gaps. The pressure to do this can be so stressful that they end up avoiding social interaction altogether. The alternative is to "be yourself," whatever that means. But being yourself in social situations can be difficult if you don't like yourself and struggle against being a shy or socially awkward individual.

TOOL FINDER You may find the compassion-focused mood repair strategies in Chapter 11 helpful as you make changes in your social interactions.

❏ **Negative communication style:** *Do you find yourself being more passive and negative—or, alternatively, more irritable and angry—in your conversations with others? Does depression affect how you talk with friends and family members?* As mentioned above, negativity gets transferred to personal communication during depressed moods. But even more than that, people who are feeling depressed tend to be more passive in conversation, to take longer pauses, to talk more slowly and with less volume, and to avoid eye contact. Family and friends will find this communication and interaction style uncomfortable, and so may try to avoid the depressed persons. What this means is that these individuals may need to become more conscious of their interaction style, and to use the social mood repair strategies to correct these maladaptive communication styles and improve their social relationships.

➤➤➤➤ Repair Strategy ㊴: Count Your Connections

The first step in reconnecting with others is to do an audit of your social support network. Who are the people you have relationships with—from casual acquaintances to intimate family members? Are there some people from your past whom you haven't contacted for a long time? Could you potentially connect with others, but have never bothered to follow up on previous conversations with them?

Use Repair Strategy 39 if . . .

- you want to begin the process of improving your social life, regardless of the barriers you have endorsed in the checklist above. To make changes, you need to know where to start. Most people consider their social relationships only when they are emotional; rarely do they assess their social networks in a more objective, nonemotional manner.

- you assume that your social network is limited because of introversion, social anxiety, or devaluation of social relationships. This strategy can be particularly informative, because it gives you a more realistic perspective on the size of your social network.

- you've neglected social relations for a long period of time and so have lost contact with several people in your life.

REPAIR STRATEGY 39 INSTRUCTIONS

1. **When you are not feeling depressed, spend some time really thinking about your relationships—not only the number of people you know, but also the quality and significance of your connections with others.** You can use the Social Network Inventory form on the facing page to help you assess your social support network. You may find it useful to take another inventory at some future date, so feel free to copy the form or print it out from *www.guilford.com/clark7-forms*.

   You will probably discover that your network of people is much larger than you realized. Also, you may be surprised at the number of people you've neglected—whose connections have worn thin because of infrequent contact. These may even be family members you've not spoken to in years, or past "best friends" you now rarely contact. In addition, think about coworkers or acquaintances you could get to know but you've never bothered to contact.

2. **The fact is that depression often drives wedges between people, separating depressed persons from loved ones. Consider the possibility that there are people whose company you used to really enjoy, but whom you've not seen for some time.** Is there a conflict between you and a close friend or family member that not only causes separation but has a negative effect on you by itself? Because you have been feeling so depressed lately, have you been neglecting, or even starving, your social support network?

In helping Suzanne complete the Social Network Inventory, her therapist helped her discover several things about her social life. First, Suzanne had far more friends than she realized, but found that she was relying too much on one or two friends for social contact. Second, she was surprised to learn that she was spending more time with people she really didn't enjoy, rather than with friends and family members who had a positive effect on her mood state. And she would never have believed that she was having so little contact with close family members who (she assumed) played key roles in her life. For Suzanne, the inventory was a stark reminder that depression had had a much greater negative effect on her social relations than she'd ever realized.

⫸➡ Repair Strategy ④⓪: Engage in Social Planning

To make changes in how you relate to others, you need to develop a plan. Taking more initiative in your social life won't happen by accident. You need to be strategic.

Social Network Inventory

Instructions: Complete this inventory over several days when you are in a positive mood state. Brainstorm a list of people you have contact with, either face to face or long distance through telephone, email, or social media. Note how often you have contact (i.e., several times a day to once or twice a year) and the approximate date of your last contact (e.g., several weeks ago). Then rate your personal level of enjoyment when associating with each person; use a scale from 0 = absolutely no enjoyment to 10 = extremely enjoyable experience. Finally, note any interpersonal problems or issues you have with each person that might affect the relationship.

Name of person	Frequency of contact (note date of last contact)	Rate enjoyment (0–10)	List any interpersonal conflicts/ issues
Family members			
Friends			
Coworkers			
Acquaintances			

Use Repair Strategy 40 if . . .

- you are introverted, are socially anxious, or devalue social relationships.
- you exhibit excessive negativity, people pleasing, reassurance seeking, or negative communication patterns.

REPAIR STRATEGY 40 INSTRUCTIONS

1. **Take a close look at the various people you've listed as family, friends, coworkers, or acquaintances on your Social Network Inventory, and engage in brainstorming to think about different ways you could make contact with these people.** In some cases you may need to increase social contact, whereas in others you may need to make new connections or reestablish long-lost contact. Take some time to brainstorm a wide range of social activities and other ways you could interact with the persons you have listed. You could begin with your spouse/partner, children, siblings, parents, and cousins, and then work down through best friends, casual friends, coworkers, and acquaintances. Contact might involve face-to-face social activities like having dinner, visiting, going to a sports event or concert, or going shopping; or it could involve Internet-based social media like Facebook, email, or Skype. The Internet has opened up previously unimaginable ways to reconnect with people who are as close as next door or who are thousands of miles away. This is your opportunity to be creative and think about all the different ways to make connections with those around you.

> **TOOL FINDER** Brainstorming is covered in Chapter 3 (Repair Strategy 10).

Suzanne's list of possible social activities included the following:

- Call my sister and see if she is available for lunch this Friday.
- Call a couple of my best friends at least twice a week.
- Create a Facebook page to reach out to some old friends I haven't seen in years.
- Email my cousin Emily in California to see if she would like to Skype.

2. **Make a list of all the ways you could engage in a range of social activities with each of the people listed in your Social Network Inventory.** You will need to be specific in your description of each social activity. Don't leave anything to guess-

work. Describe exactly what you could do, when, and with whom. For close family and friends, more intense social contact (such as a dinner invitation) might be appropriate, whereas something less intense (like an email or a short phone call) might be appropriate for someone you've not seen for a while. The important thing is to create a plan and chart a course for improving your relationships with others.

> Taking the initiative to create social opportunities with others will reduce anxiety and awkwardness by putting you in control of the social interaction.

3. **Consult this list of possible social activities when you are feeling down or depressed; select an individual; and then put into motion a fairly easy social activity that you have listed for this individual.** Do something, even a small gesture like an email or phone call, to make a connection when you are feeling depressed. You will find this a particularly powerful mood repair strategy.

➤ Repair Strategy ㊶: Learn to Listen

The amount of enjoyment you get from social interactions depends as much on your interpersonal style as it does on your social companion and what you are doing. That is, the potential for mood repair increases when you have an enjoyable, pleasant social interaction. One way to ensure such a positive experience is to practice good interpersonal skills. And one of the very best social skills is *listening*. Most of us find listening hard to do, and this is especially true when we are feeling depressed. We are much more likely to talk about ourselves than to listen to a friend or family member.

Good listening is called *reflective listening*. It involves actively listening to what the other person is saying, making appropriate eye contact, nodding that you understand what is being said, and paraphrasing what you are hearing. Rather than giving advice, telling the person what to do, or talking about yourself, you are simply communicating to the other person that you understand, and that you have empathy and concern for his/her issue. Reflective listening has an immediate payoff: People love to be heard, to feel that another person is interested in their situation. If you add questions to reflective listening—well-placed questions that again show genuine attention and interest—you will find that others will want to be around you. They will want to socialize with you because they will find you a warm and receptive person.

> Building good listening skills is imperative to building high-quality personal relationships.

You may be thinking that it is impossible to learn to be a good listener or to show interest in other people by asking questions about their lives. Nothing could be further from the truth. After 25 years of training clinical psychologists, I can tell you that our students do not start out as good listeners. In their very first year of training, my colleagues and I spend considerable time teaching these young people how to listen. Reflective listening is a skill you too can learn if you want, but you have to be intentional in doing this.

Are you a good listener? If you are struggling in your relationships with others, could poor listening be one of your problems? Although some people seem to be natural-born listeners, most of us have to learn listening skills. Most people find talking about themselves quite automatic and maybe quite enjoyable; it's much harder to focus on other people and listen to their stories. I have a friend who is an excellent listener. He looks at you when you're speaking, nods appropriately, smiles, asks questions, and seems genuinely interested. I have noticed that other men in particular love to be around him. They enjoy his company and seek him out to join them in social activities. He's popular because he's a good listener, easygoing, and flexible. So practice your listening skills.

Use Repair Strategy 41 if your social barriers include . . .

- negative beliefs about others.

- excessive negativity in general.

- blaming others.

- negative communication style.

REPAIR STRATEGY 41 INSTRUCTIONS

1. **Start by "practicing" on a close friend or family member. You could admit, "I am trying to be a better listener, so as we have this conversation, I will be intentionally trying out a few communication skills. I'd like your opinion on how I am doing when we're through."**

2. **After several practice sessions, begin using your reflective listening and questioning skills in natural conversation with family and friends.** Since reflective listening is an important characteristic of good communication, it will improve the quality of your social contacts with people. And forming better connections with people is a potent pathway to depressive mood repair. You will feel better about yourself as you become better at expressing genuine interest in other people's lives.

➤➤ Repair Strategy ㊷: Initiate Interpersonal Contact

Most people who struggle with low mood find it easier to be passive, submissive, and unassertive in their social relationships than to initiate contact with others. So taking the initiative, being more assertive, and making the first move to engage in social interchanges may seem exceedingly difficult, especially if you are also an introverted person or you're battling social anxiety as well as depression. But, in fact, waiting for friends or family to make contact means that you're not in control of your social life. It puts you in a more vulnerable and helpless state, and deprives you of the opportunity to use social contact to repair your depressed mood. Although the prospect may seem intimidating to you, the only way to reenergize your connections with others is to take the lead and initiate social contact.

I will assume that initiating contact is something you've already realized is important, but that you avoid or postpone it for any number of reasons. Nevertheless, fear of doing something that is uncomfortable is not a good reason for continuing to depend on others to take the first step. It may actually surprise and please acquaintances and family members if you start inviting them to do something with you.

Use Repair Strategy 42 if . . .

- you are introverted or socially anxious.
- you are a people pleaser who tends to be submissive and unassertive.
- you are suspicious of others, and so you struggle with trust issues.
- you are fearful of being hurt by others.

REPAIR STRATEGY 42 INSTRUCTIONS

1. Identify one or two familiar friends with whom you are comfortable, and start by initiating social contact with them.

2. Use a communication medium you are comfortable with, whether this is email, text messaging, voice mail, or a simple phone call.

3. Suggest a social activity that is brief and time-limited, such as having coffee together or going out to lunch.

4. Allow the person the opportunity to suggest times for social contact that might be convenient for him/her.

5. Begin taking the social initiative when you are in a more positive mood state, and then gradually work toward doing this when you are feeling more depressed.

6. Gradually increase the complexity of the social activity to include contacts that may be more challenging, such as hosting a dinner party.

Phoning friends and asking them out to lunch caused Suzanne considerable anxiety, because she was so concerned she would be considered an unwanted intrusion into their busy lives. So she started by calling her two sisters in the evening, because she knew that they liked to have phone conversations. She then decided to email a couple of friends about going out to lunch, which she felt was a less pressured way to initiate contact. Finally, she invited to dinner a couple of friends she had not seen in a while. This was, however, a much more threatening social initiative, so she started with the phone calls to her sisters and gradually worked her way up to the more difficult initiatives.

▸▸▸▸ Repair Strategy ㊸: Practice Being a Greeter

If you've been feeling depressed for a while, it is likely that you've stopped being a friendly person. No doubt you tend to ignore people, to go about your daily activities alone, and to avoid eye contact or interaction with others as much as possible. But saying hello, smiling, asking acquaintances or even strangers about their day—that is, offering friendly greetings—has a positive influence on others and will actually make you feel better. A smile or casual remark to the many strangers you interact with on a daily basis, such as cashiers, store clerks, waiters, people waiting for an elevator, delivery persons, or people waiting in line at a restaurant, expresses friendliness. Even though you may not feel like being friendly, these small behaviors can have a momentary positive effect on your mood state.

We all differ greatly in our personalities, and friendliness may be much more difficult for you than it is for others. At first it will feel odd and quite phony, but with repetition it will come to feel more genuine.

Use Repair Strategy 43 if your social barriers include . . .

- excessive negativity.
- fear of getting hurt.
- blaming others.
- irritated communication style.

REPAIR STRATEGY 43 INSTRUCTIONS

1. **Start your friendliness training by expressing social gestures that are less threatening for you.** Practice saying hello to people, smiling at them, making eye contact, being courteous, holding the door to let others go through first, or mak-

ing a positive comment about a person's service toward you (such as a salesperson who has helped you find a store item). In other words, turn from grumpiness to friendliness in your daily social interactions. When you do this, you will find that even this change in very basic interpersonal behavior will have a positive mood repair effect.

2. **Then try simple conversation. Make a variety of common remarks to express casual interest and friendliness when you are in contact with strangers:**

- Ask, "How's your day going?"

- Comment on the weather.

- If you are waiting, offer a sympathetic remark to others about the long line or wait time.

- If a person is accompanied by a baby or pet, think of something complimentary to say.

- Make a positive comment about the person's clothing or appearance.

> **Acting friendly counters negative mood; being grumpy intensifies negativity.**

- If the person is carrying grocery bags, make a remark about shopping.

⫸ Repair Strategy 44: Take the Intimacy Initiative

The majority of us have loved ones in our lives; we have partners, children, grandchildren, parents, and/or siblings. We are all part of some family network, even though members of this family may be spread across the country or around the world. Fortunately, our global communications systems now make it possible for us to maintain steady contact with loved ones, regardless of their geographic distance from us. So it is unlikely that any actual barrier to communication with our loved ones is keeping us apart. Conflict, procrastination, or sheer neglect is much more likely to be causing any separation from them. Strong intimate connections can do wonders to repair the sense of abandonment and alienation that can result from being stuck in the blues.

Use Repair Strategy 44 when . . .

- you've slipped into neglecting or underestimating the value of relationships.

- you are angry with someone close to you.

- you are blaming others.

- you are fearful of getting hurt again.

REPAIR STRATEGY 44 INSTRUCTIONS

1. **Go back and review your Social Network Inventory, focusing on the amount of time you've spent with your immediate family members or other loved ones.** Have you been neglecting your loved ones for work or other pursuits? Are you spending regular "quality time" with your partner, children, or parents? Are you missing opportunities to connect with the people most important in your life? When you are with your family members, are you showing real interest in their lives, or are you preoccupied with your own personal issues? Do you take the initiative in doing positive interpersonal activities, or are members of your family isolated from each other, spending all their time on screens (watching TV, surfing the Internet, texting, Facebooking, etc.)? In regard to your partner, when was the last time you were intimate—that you took the initiative in being intimate, or even expressed love and appreciation? Are there conflicts or misunderstandings that need to be dealt with to heal a relationship? When was the last time you really showed you cared about the loved ones in your life? As you can see, there is a host of reasons why you may not be as close as you might be to your partner or other family members. Feeling depressed can separate you from loved ones, mainly through neglect, avoidance, loss of interest, passivity, and/or waiting for others to take the initiative.

2. **If you decide after reviewing your inventory that you have been neglecting or pulling away from your family members, make a plan by outlining some specific ways you can reconnect with loved ones.** Remember, it is up to you to take the initiative and make time for your partner and family. You need to give them the message that you want to spend time with them, that you are still interested in their lives. It is also important that you express some love, care, and closeness to your loved ones, which is the topic of the next chapter. So I encourage you to take the time to reconnect with your loved ones. It's an investment in time that will pay off in big returns toward repairing the loneliness and despair you may be feeling during those times when you are stuck in the blues.

3. **After spending some time with a loved one, reflect on its effect on your emotional well-being.** How did you feel while you were with your loved one? Were you able to express and receive love and affection from this person? How has the opportunity for intimacy made you feel about yourself and life more generally? Does intimacy have a positive or negative effect on your depressive mood state? It is important to be realistic and balanced in your evaluation. Try to determine how you really feel after being intimate, and not how you think you should feel.

Intimacy is not a panacea for all misery. It is quite possible that you struggle with intimacy, or that you have serious relationship problems with your partner or another loved one. For example, people who have been abused may find intimacy counterproductive or even actively harmful. In such cases, it is important to seek professional help to deal with these issues.

⟫⟫⟫ Repair Strategy ㊺: Be a Joiner, Not an Avoider

One of the main social causes for the increase in depression and anxiety in contemporary society is the loss of community. Because of our increased mobility, we are often cut off from family and neighbors. Most of us live in sprawling urban or suburban communities, where we hardly know our neighbors and have reduced our involvement in community organizations (religious congregations, charitable organizations, political parties, and the like). Many people live isolated lives devoid of any meaningful sense of community. However, there are many potential communities all around you, and becoming a member of one or two of these communities can be a great way to repair depressed mood.

The variety of groups open to new members is almost endless. There are book clubs, hobby groups, social action groups, volunteer and charitable organizations, faith groups (churches, synagogues, mosques, etc.), exercise and stress reduction groups (yoga, Pilates, etc.), university extracurricular courses, and numerous others. Whatever your interest, there is probably a class or group of people who share your interest. And because these groups are formed around interests that bring like-minded individuals together, they are great ways to meet people. If you find it difficult to initiate conversations, joining an exercise class or a book club makes it easier, because you can talk about the group's interest or common task. Of course, going to a new group for the first time can be quite intimidating, but groups that are open to new members are used to new people and usually know how to make people feel welcome. After attending three or four group meetings, you will feel more comfortable, but you do have to give yourself time to settle into the group.

I can't stress enough how important it is to belong to a community that is more than just your place of employment. If you are spending every evening and weekend alone, with no involvement with other people, then you will feel depressed. Even if you have a busy work schedule, travel a lot, or have an active family, you need to make your own connections with others through some form of community involvement.

Use Repair Strategy 45 if your social barriers include . . .

- fear of getting hurt or of being negatively evaluated by others.
- self-initiated pressure; that is, you feel you have to be someone you're not.

REPAIR STRATEGY 45 INSTRUCTIONS

1. **Begin by identifying your own personal interests, such as sports, a hobby, education, religion, or social activism.** Reviewing some of the work you did in the Chapter 9 exercises on goals and values may help you identify your interests.

2. **Then search your local newspaper, community bulletin boards, local university, or municipal library; conduct a Google search of your community; or contact the local parks and recreation department for information on groups in your community.**

3. **Once you have identified a group that matches one of your interests, muster the courage and go to the first group meeting.** It will be difficult and anxiety-provoking at first, but the potential payoff in reducing feelings of loneliness and depression can be enormous. Many of these groups engage in social action, such as raising money for medical research or assisting less fortunate people in your community. As discussed in the next chapter, helping others through charitable organizations is an especially good way to counter depressed mood.

4. **Give yourself a chance to acclimate to the group.** Most people feel conspicuous and uncomfortable when they first attend a group. Of course, some people feel more uncomfortable than others, but it is probably more common than not to feel ill at ease. Therefore, it is important to give yourself time to get accustomed to the group. You don't have to participate at the beginning; give yourself time to determine the group members' ability to accept you and your own ability to accept them. There will be some members of the group you really like and others you will find difficult, maybe even obnoxious. But learning to tolerate diversity is important, and you don't have to perform for the group; that is, you don't have to be chatty and convivial if that's not your personality. Instead, be yourself, and give yourself and the group time to warm up to each other. Don't quit after one meeting, but go back several times to really give yourself a chance to determine whether this group is for you.

Suzanne was already involved in her synagogue, but now that she was retired from her teaching job, she had a lot more free time on her hands. So she needed to expand her community involvement. She heard that a retired English professor was leading a women's book club she thought might be interesting, so she obtained the contact information and called the group leader to see whether they were accepting new members. It turned out that the group was full at the moment, but a couple of women were planning to move to other cities over the summer, and the group leader thought there would be openings in a month or two. So Suzanne put her name on a waiting list and was able to join the group several weeks later. She also joined the local chapter of the American Association of Retired Persons (AARP) and became a frequent reader of the AARP website (*www.aarp.org*), which she found was a great source of information. Suzanne was surprised to discover so many active people her own age who were fully engaged in community life.

Like Suzanne, you can become a member of an active community group, but you have to make the first move. So what's stopping you? If you say you don't have time, are you also saying you don't have time to look after your mental health—to do something constructive to repair your depression and enrich your life? If what's holding you up is fear or anxiety, then take the time to break out and confront your anxieties. Become a joiner and not an avoider.

⋙➤ Repair Strategy ㊻: Adopt a Four-Legged Friend

Sophie had struggled for 30 years with bipolar disorder. Although it was controlled to a certain extent by mood-stabilizing medication, Sophie still experienced occasional mood swings. At times she became manic and irrational, but more often she would fall into deep depression. After 25 years of marriage, Sophie's husband finally moved out, leaving her alone in the house. Unfortunately, Sophie had great difficulty in social situations because of her psychiatric condition, and so she spent much of her time alone at home. She didn't have paid employment, and a support worker came in to help with the housework once a week. Consequently, Sophie had a lot of free time on her hands. However, one bright spot in her life was her Maltese dog, Charlie. Charlie was 11 years old, and a strong attachment had developed between him and Sophie. Charlie expressed unconditional love toward Sophie, and because of his needs for exercise and the outdoors, Sophie would walk Charlie twice a day. It got her out of the house, and because the dog was so cute, people would often stop and ask Sophie about Charlie.

Sophie treated Charlie like a child, which was helpful, because it often seemed as if there was no one else in her life.

> **Could a pet bring greater joy and connectedness into your life?**

If you have an introverted personality or a fear of getting hurt by others, you might find that having a pet is a good starting point for making connections. However, we can't get all of our need for social interaction from our pets, so it will be important to use the other social repair strategies in this chapter to improve connections with family and friends. Also, "pet therapy" is not for everyone, so this strategy is more selective than the others discussed previously. You should consider this option only if you have an interest in and love for animals, and if your living arrangements are conducive to having a pet.

REPAIR STRATEGY 46 INSTRUCTIONS

1. **Consider whether you have the resources for a pet.** Begin by determining whether your personal living arrangements would allow you to acquire a pet. Do you live in a home or apartment that is pet-friendly? Are other members of your family interested in having a pet? Do you have the time to care for a pet? There are many practical considerations to take into account before adding a pet to your life.

2. **Determine your animal interest.** Many different types of animals are kept as pets. Dogs are extremely popular pets because of their relational quality. Since we are talking about creating a social connection to your pet, a dog (or, to a lesser extent, a cat) will be preferable. But there are many different dog and cat breeds. You should consult a breeder or veterinarian for advice on matching a breed to your particular interests and personality.

3. **Talk to a pet owner.** Talk to your friends or family members who have pets about their experiences. If you are considering a particular breed, it would be best to speak to someone who has that type of animal. You want to be fully informed about the animal's temperament before you acquire the animal as your pet.

4. **Offer to "pet-sit" an animal of the type you are considering for your pet.** If you have a friend or family member with a pet of the variety you are considering, offer to walk it or look after it over the weekend. Acquire some experience with the animal, so that you have some first-hand knowledge of what it is like to have around.

5. **Acquire your pet.** Finally, make a decision to acquire your pet, but give yourself and the animal plenty of time to adjust. It will take both of you several weeks to get adjusted to each other, so don't give up too soon. Each year thousands of animals are left at animal shelters because people give up on their pets too soon. Be patient with yourself and your animal. Note whether you are having times of enjoyment interacting with your pet.

Pets are a great source of enjoyment and connectedness for millions of people. There is little doubt that having pets improves mental and emotional health for large numbers of people. In fact, my own university recently introduced a "pet therapy" program for stressed-out students. For a couple of weeks around each exam period, local pet owners volunteer to bring their pets to the university, where students can spend a short time interacting with their cats or dogs. Even this brief and limited contact with pets has proven beneficial in reducing stress and improving mood for many of the students.

Again, being a pet owner is not for everyone, because considerable work and responsibility is involved in looking after an animal. Nevertheless, if you love animals or once had a pet, introducing a pet into your life could boost your mood. Having a pet is often particularly helpful for people who have lost a loved one. We all need opportunities to express and receive love and affection; a pet can play an important part in fulfilling this need.

Losing a pet can also trigger depressed mood that may last for weeks. Although you may be reluctant to acquire a new pet after you have lost a beloved animal, it is probably important that you give yourself time to grieve for your loss and then introduce a new pet into your life. If you've never had a pet, consider whether one would be helpful in dealing with your depressed mood and loneliness. Having a pet can be an important part of your mood repair strategy.

Getting Connected

For human beings, relationships are critical for survival. Unfortunately, depression can undermine your desire and ability to establish connections with others. Depending on the depth and duration of your depression, overcoming your barriers to social connectedness and breaking your automatic tendency to withdraw and avoid others may prove challenging. Although it will take persistence on your part, you can make significant improvements in both your mood and your social life by using the mood repair strategies in this chapter. In fact, many psychologists believe that improving relationships is the single most important way to overcome depression. There is even a type of treatment called *interpersonal psychotherapy* that focuses exclusively on relationships—and it is one of only a handful of psychological interventions shown to be effective for treating clinical depression.[2]

Our highly urbanized and technologically integrated society creates both barriers and opportunities to expanding our social support networks. The digital world makes it possible for us to live completely isolated, singular lives, even while swimming in a sea of humanity. But at the same time, Internet-based social media and the tools for using them (smartphones and similar devices) allow us to make connections with friends and loved ones living practically anywhere in the world. Geographic distance is no longer a barrier to relationships. So don't ignore or minimize the positive effects of your digital connectedness. Creating relationships with others may be the most important way to overcome your feelings of loneliness and despair.

TOOL FINDER ■ If you believe that other people don't like you, that you'll never be accepted, or that you just don't have the ability to connect with others, use the cognitive mood repair strategies in Chapter 4 to change the way you think about yourself and others. You may need to do this work before you can use the social change strategies described in this chapter.

- If you are caught in depressive rumination, or convinced that there is nothing you can do about your isolation from others while you are depressed, review Chapter 6.

- If you are feeling hopeless about the future, or questioning whether there is any sense in even trying to improve your social life, consult Chapter 9 on life goals and values.

- You may have known for some time that you need to reconnect with people, but you've been procrastinating and have avoided taking the initiative. If so, Chapter 13, which discusses ways of breaking procrastination and other avoidance patterns, will help you deal with this problem.

- Finally, you may be feeling that you don't have the motivation or energy to deal with people. If low energy or fatigue is a problem for you, see Chapter 12 on physical exercise, sleep, and diet. It may be that you need to work on these issues first to restore your activity level, so you'll feel more engaged with life and more prepared to participate in social activities.

11 express kindness and compassion

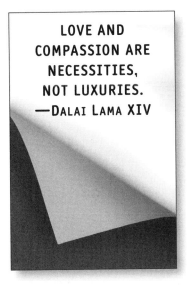

> LOVE AND COMPASSION ARE NECESSITIES, NOT LUXURIES.
> —DALAI LAMA XIV

Love has occupied the center stage of human literature, drama, philosophy, religion, and storytelling for centuries. There is a universal recognition that *compassionate love*—that is, our ability to show kindness and sympathy to ourselves and to others—is a central ingredient of the fulfilled, enriched life. The positive effects of such love are enduring, affecting both the givers and receivers of the acts it inspires.

The Biblical adage "It is more blessed to give than to receive" (Acts 20:35) has been experienced and witnessed by all of us. A friend diagnosed with cancer continued to volunteer at the local soup kitchen throughout her chemotherapy, helping her withstand a difficult regimen and sustain hope. A woman in my practice spoke about how her volunteer work at the hospital brought a sense of meaning and purpose to her life while she was mourning the loss of her husband. A woman who had suffered for many years at the hands of a violent husband now devotes her life to helping other victims of domestic violence, describing this work as having healing effects on her. A young man explained to me the sense of despair he felt while undergoing cancer treatment, and yet, after beating the odds and surviving his catastrophic illness, he experienced a renewed interest in and concern for the plight of others. And then there was the pastor who suffered from repeated periods of depression, but found that acts of ministering to the needs of others helped lift him out of the depression trap.

Compassion is contagious in the best possible sense: It has a positive impact on the emotions of all it touches. Unfortunately, depressed mood makes it difficult to give compassion to others, and even more so to ourselves. When we are feeling low, our attention typically becomes self-focused in a negative way, as we ruminate about feeling so sad and wonder why we can't grope our way out of the darkness. Depression's cycle of negativity and self-criticism can cause us to shrink into our own small worlds, preventing us from experiencing the peace and joy that come from exercising compassion.

The strategies in this chapter can help you widen your perspective and extend love and kindness to yourself and others. When you're trapped by sadness, you may feel that you don't deserve compassion or cannot extend it to others. But in the same way that conventional wisdom says you have to take care of your own health if you are to have the strength to care for others, it's important to learn self-compassion. The purpose of this chapter is to explain how you can develop a *compassionate mind*, because this steady state will help you repair your mood before it drags you too far down.

Use compassion-focused strategies if your depressive mood is characterized by . . .

- negative thinking that is highly self-critical, maybe even bordering on self-loathing or hatred.

- impatience, frustration, or anger with yourself or others.

- depressive rumination.

- loss of peace and contentment.

- self-centeredness involving a preoccupation with your current state and problems.

The Compassionate Mind

Compassion is a little like a "sixth sense." We all recognize compassion but struggle to define it, let alone understand it. The *merriam-webster.com* definition—"sympathetic consciousness of others' distress together with a desire to alleviate it"—is a good starting point, but hardly enough to help us develop the compassionate mind that can repair mood. We need to drill down deeper into the concept of compassion, especially self-compassion, to unlock its potential to overcome depressed mood.

Compassion is such an essential part of humanity that it's not an overstatement to say it is critical to survival itself. As a species, our ability to survive has depended in large part on

> Compassion is the glue of humanity; it binds us together as families and communities that have ensured the survival of the species.

the protection gained from forming groups (extended family groups, tribes, etc.) and being able to care for our young through their many years of dependency on adults. Getting along with each other and caring for our young require compassion. Without compassion, our species would become extinct, just as we all individually experience an "inner death" when we lack compassion.

The sidebar "The Compassionate Brain" on the next page describes one theory of how the brain uses an innate capacity for compassion to regulate emotions and prevent us from spiraling into depression. The diagram below illustrates the emotion regulation sequence of compassion, showing that *self*-soothing must come before we can care for others, which in turn produces feelings of peace and contentment. The compassionate mind, which has the power to repair mood, is maintained through this rejuvenating pathway.

> **Exercise a caregiving mentality to create a brain state of calm and peace.**

Maintaining a compassionate mind has clear benefits for all of us. But what exactly makes up the compassionate mind? What qualities do we need to develop to experience compassion as a steady state and thereby mitigate depressed feelings? According to Paul Gilbert, the compassionate mind consists of . . .

- an appreciation for life—the ability to experience joy in simply being alive.
- valuing relationships or connection with others.
- sensitivity to the needs and emotions of self and others.
- deep awareness and empathy toward human suffering in self and others.
- a desire to express patience and generosity toward those in pain and suffering.
- increased tolerance of distress.
- psychological-mindedness—heightened awareness of human nature.
- an accepting, nonjudgmental attitude.

THE IMPORTANCE OF TOLERATING THE HUMAN EXPERIENCE OF PAIN

As can be seen from the list above, recognizing others' suffering and being moved to help, *without* fear or repugnance toward the natural human experience of pain, is an

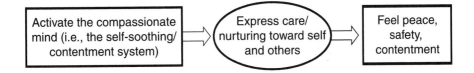

the compassionate brain

British psychologist Paul Gilbert has spent the last 30 years researching the nature of compassion, its evolution within the human species, and the development of a specialized form of cognitive behavior therapy for anxiety and depression called *compassion-focused therapy*.[1] In his book *The Compassionate Mind,* Gilbert argues that compassion not only is fundamental to human evolution, but is "hard-wired" into the human brain. To understand how this works, he suggests that we regulate our emotions through three interrelated brain systems:

- The *incentive/resource* system motivates us to seek out resources that aid in our survival, assure our prosperity, and maintain our status within society. It fuels ambition and helps us reach our goals, but in overdrive it can leave us perpetually dissatisfied as we relentlessly strive for more. It may push us too far with the help of dopamine, the neurotransmitter implicated in the reward centers of the brain.

- The *threat/self-protection* system warns us of danger, activating feelings of anxiety, fear, anger, or disgust. Centered in the primitive brain structure called the amygdala, it powers our fight-or-flight response and thus protects us from life-threatening situations. However, when overactivated for longer periods of time, it triggers the release of the stress hormone cortisol to a degree that can be harmful to health. In depression, the threat/protection system may be responsible for our desire to withdraw into a self-protective mode of existence.

- The *soothing/contentment* system brings a sense of safety, peace, and connection with self and others. It involves nurturance, empathy, and validation. When the incentive system pushes us too hard and the self-protection system becomes *over*protective, this system can step in to release endorphins and the hormone oxytocin, which comfort and relax us, like the soothing effects of a hot cup of tea (insert here your favorite beverage!) while enjoying the warmth of a roaring fire on a cold winter's evening.

According to Gilbert, being compassionate brings balance to our emotions by activating the self-soothing brain state, which then counters the excesses of the incentive and threat brain systems.

important part of compassion. When I first started work as a psychologist, a young woman was referred to me who had suffered a spinal cord injury resulting in quadriplegia. I was so distraught over her incredible disability and suffering that I was barely able to offer her the psychological services she needed. Have you ever lost a loved one and then had friends and acquaintances practically ignore you? They may have been prevented from expressing compassion toward you because they felt anxious about or uncomfortable with your loss. Compassionate people are able to tolerate the pain and suffering of others. This is an essential precondition to expressing compassion and loving kindness toward others.

> An ability to accept and tolerate human pain and suffering in self and others is a prerequisite for exercising compassion.

TOOL FINDER The strategies for achieving acceptance and mindfulness, discussed in Chapter 7, are helpful in developing tolerance to pain and suffering in self and others.

FIRST COMES SELF-COMPASSION

Another facet of the compassionate mind illustrated in the diagram is probably less obvious to most people: To express loving kindness and compassion to others, you first must have the capacity to act compassionately toward yourself. If you are bound up by self-criticism, regrets, and negativity, you won't be able to extend yourself outward to the needs of others. All of your personal resources—your time, energy, and effort—will be consumed by self-focus, rumination, and maybe even self-pity. There will be nothing left for friends, family, or community. This is not to say it's impossible to be compassionate and also self-critical. It's just that the extremes of self-criticism often found in more severe depressive moods can siphon off the motivation and energy required to be caring toward others.

An ability to engage in self-compassion is the cornerstone of the mood repair strategies discussed in this chapter; it can contribute directly to recovery from depressed mood. For this reason, a lot of emphasis is placed on self-compassion in the following mood repair strategies.

Self-compassion is not an obvious concept. It means being open, understanding, and accepting

> Negative mood repair occurs through self-compassion, acceptance, and tolerance.

of our painful experiences, so that we develop a deep empathy and tolerance for our feelings and difficulties.[1] Kristin Neff, of the University of Texas at Austin, has identified three basic components to self-compassion:[2]

1. Kindness and understanding toward yourself, rather than self-criticism and judgment (e.g., "I'm tolerant of my own flaws and inadequacies").

2. The capacity to view negative personal experiences as part of the larger human experience, rather than as separate and isolating events (e.g., "I try to see my failings as part of the human condition").

3. The ability to hold painful thoughts and feelings in balanced awareness, rather than in overidentification (e.g., "When I fail at something important to me, I try to keep things in perspective").

Do not confuse self-compassion with self-pity or selfishness. Self-compassion is a self-focused sympathy, an emotional openness to your own suffering. By contrast, self-pity is overidentifying with the victim role, and/or having a sense of angry injustice in which you see yourself as "poor me" and complain or become tearful about your situation.[1] Instead, self-compassion means that you develop a patient understanding of yourself. For example, let's say you are feeling hurt by some angry, unkind remarks from your spouse—but as you reflect on that negative feeling, you realize you've gotten through it before, with more endurance and courage than you expected. Moreover, selfishness involves a disconnection from others: It involves putting your personal needs ahead of others' needs, or becoming so engrossed in your own problems that you become consumed by your emotional reactions, and thereby find it difficult to adopt a more objective, distant perspective.

You might think of the difference between self-compassion and self-pity as akin to the difference between art and pornography. We all know the difference when we see it, but it can be difficult to articulate. I had an elderly relative who epitomized self-pity rather than self-compassion. He complained constantly about his physical ailments, going through each ache and pain in excruciating detail, totally consumed by his own situation. Eventually he died at 84 years of age, still complaining and looking for sympathy from others. It was awfully hard to give in to his requests; my family and I could feel our "compassion meters" quickly plunge to zero.

In the end, self-compassion, unlike self-pity, involves acceptance of whatever our state may be at a given moment. As noted in Chapter 4, we are often the harshest critics of ourselves. So when we learn acceptance, tolerance, and patience with ourselves, we are in a better position to extend this attitude toward others.

THE DEPRESSIVE MIND VERSUS THE COMPASSIONATE MIND

Being stuck in the blues undermines compassion, for two main reasons:

1. *Overfocusing on ourselves promotes self-pity.* During low moods we automatically withdraw into ourselves, becoming highly focused on our own difficulties, issues, and emotional state. The threat/self-protection emotion system in the brain becomes activated, so that all of our attention is focused on "me." This excessive self-focused attention limits our ability to adopt a more objective, accepting approach to our situation, leaving us vulnerable to drifting into self-pity rather than self-compassion. If all we can think about are our personal problems, then we are not thinking about the difficulties faced by others.

2. *Extreme negativity promotes self-blame.* When feeling depressed, we do not see the world or ourselves clearly. We adopt a highly negative, often critical, blaming, and hopeless outlook, especially toward ourselves. This negativity distorts our perspective, reinforces giving up, and prevents us from expressing any degree of kindness to self or others. We become immobilized—unable to accept the current situation, but at the same time incapable of moving forward.

> **TOOL FINDER**   Chapters 4 and 6 offer strategies for replacing the highly negative, self-critical attitudes of depressed mood with an outlook that cultivates the compassionate mind.

Negativity makes it difficult to accept ourselves and our problems; it thwarts forward movement, leaving us truly stuck in the blues.

You don't have to remain stuck in self-pity, unable to move forward in your life. You can use the compassion-focused repair strategies described below to bring patience, kindness, and acceptance to yourself, your current situation, and your interactions with others.

➤➤➤ Repair Strategy 47:
Practice Intentional Appreciation

Most of us go through our daily lives focusing on the various work and family responsibilities that are uppermost in our minds. We can become so preoccupied with our personal agendas that we are completely oblivious of all the small delights in life that bring us even a momentary degree of comfort, peace, and calm. Examples of such small, brief comforts might include waking up in a warm comfortable bed, taking a soothing shower, having that first sip of freshly brewed coffee, taking a first taste of your favorite food, looking out on a scenic view, sitting on your deck on a warm spring morning, or listening to your favorite music. How many of these small comforts are bestowed on us throughout the day without our noticing them? Have you been feeling so down, so preoccupied with personal difficulties, that you haven't even noticed—let alone appreciated—the small comforts in life? You know the old adage "Stop and smell the roses." Gilbert calls this "developing the art of appreciation."[1]

> **Are you missing out on all the small comforts happening in your daily life?**

If being busy and preoccupied with your worries and difficulties can drag down your mood, then shifting your attention to the small comforts that are happening in your life will have the opposite effect: It will improve your mood, at least momentarily. The moment is what we are working on—taking life one moment at a time. If you are thinking that you have no small pleasures, or that no comforting moments are happening in your life, you've likely been too busy and preoccupied to notice. You need to learn to slow down, to shift your attention so you can "stop and smell the roses." This is actually a powerful strategy for repairing negative mood.

> **TOOL FINDER**   Chapters 2 and 5 have presented record-keeping exercises to track positive or pleasurable experiences in your daily life—activities that are associated with a small degree of happiness. You can use the same approach to develop the art of appreciation by slightly modifying the focus.

Use Repair Strategy 47 if you're . . .

- stuck in the blues; you are convinced that nothing good is happening in your life.
- caught in depressive rumination; your mind is filled with misery and difficulty.
- convinced there is no comfort in your life, only misery and disappointment.
- stressed out or overwhelmed by life's demands.

REPAIR STRATEGY 47 INSTRUCTIONS

1. Over a 3- to 5-day period, why not be intentional and make a list of all the little things, the minor experiences throughout your day that bring a small,

momentary degree of calm and peace to your life? You can use the partial Small Pleasures Record below as a template for this exercise, or print out a complete copy of this form from *www.guilford.com/clark7-forms*. Enter these pleasurable experiences in the left column of the form.

2. **In addition to capturing these brief moments of peace and comfort, learn to pay attention to and appreciate what other people are doing for you.** Think about the person who holds the elevator for you, the coworker who brings you a cup of coffee, the friend who asks about your day, a stranger who makes a friendly remark, a waiter who provides good service, a retail clerk with whom you have a polite exchange. These small acts of kindness and goodness probably happen to you throughout your day, but how often do you take notice? Can you imagine the positive effect on your mood, your outlook on life, if you shifted your attention from the negative or even mean behavior of others to the acts of human goodness all around you? Taking in the goodness of humanity, including the personal acts of caring and soothing that come your way from others, can have a profound impact on repairing your negative mood. Enter these small kindnesses in the right column of the Small Pleasures Record.

Dennis returned from a combat tour in Afghanistan an angry, cynical, and depressed person. For the first time in his life, he experienced intense bouts of depressed mood; during these times, he would withdraw into his "man cave," watch videos for hours, and drink. These times of withdrawal were becoming more and more frequent, and his family learned not to interrupt his "down time." But withdrawal was not Dennis's only problem. His interactions with people at work, at home, and elsewhere became more and more strained. He seemed irritable, impatient, and short-

Small Pleasures Record

Calming, peaceful, pleasurable momentary experiences	Small expressions of kindness and caring by others
1.	1.
2.	2.

tempered with practically everyone with whom he came into contact. Dennis's entire focus throughout the day was on all the stupid, ignorant, selfish things that he perceived in others. How people drove, what they said to him, how they acted—all Dennis could see was human ignorance, and this filled him with contempt for humanity. This angry, negative, cynical outlook did nothing but feed his anger and depression.

Working with Dennis to help him shift gears and begin to take notice of the goodness in others, to focus on instances of momentary peace and calm, was an enormous challenge. His view was "How could I possibly buy into this crap after all the suffering, cruelty, and stupidity I saw in Afghanistan?" It took Dennis a long time even to consider the potential personal benefit he could experience from working on the art of appreciation. Learning to see how others valued and cared for him, while also appreciating momentary experiences of peace and calm, helped lift him out of dysphoria, discouragement, and despair.

⯈⯈⯈⯈ Repair Strategy ㊽: Build a Compassionate Image

When you think of "perfect" kindness and compassion, does an image of a particular person who captures these virtues come to mind? I have several of these images: clients who have taken responsibility for significant failures or disappointments in their lives, but can forgive themselves, learn from their mistakes, and then move on with their lives. Is there someone in your own life (now or in the past), or possibly some great religious or spiritual leader, who embodies for you this notion of compassion to self and others? To adopt a compassionate mind, it is helpful to have a sense, an image of compassion. You need to be able to see active compassion toward self and others in your mind's eye. It will be difficult, if not impossible, to develop a compassionate mind without some goal—some idea or image of what you would be like if you exercised compassion and kindness toward yourself and others.

> **TOOL FINDER**   Chapter 9 has discussed the use of imagery to create a more hopeful outlook for the future (see Repair Strategy 37). The same approach can be used to create an image of the compassionate self.

Use Repair Strategy 48 when . . .

- you're being especially hard on yourself, because you are stuck in a vicious cycle of regret, self-blame, and criticism.
- you need a reminder that self-focused negativity only drives a person further into

despair, and that loving kindness, compassion, and forgiveness can be a "healing balm" to your tormented spirit.

REPAIR STRATEGY 48 INSTRUCTIONS

1. **Start with an ideal image of self-compassion. What are the characteristics, the qualities you envision when you think about a compassionate person?** Psychologist Christopher Germer, in his book *The Mindful Path to Self-Compassion,* warns that "the most difficult person in the world to hold in loving awareness is usually oneself" (p. 149). Most of us don't spend much time thinking about our good qualities, because we think this encourages pride and conceit. You may recall some version of the Biblical verse "Pride goes before destruction, a haughty spirit before a fall" (Proverbs 16:18), and so you may fear that dwelling on your good points might encourage misfortune. For most people struggling with depression, however, the greater problem is self-loathing. In their negativity and self-criticalness, they can become so focused on their faults, mistakes, and weaknesses that they don't see any goodness in themselves. This, of course, will make it extremely difficult to form an image of loving kindness toward themselves. And yet having an image of self-compassion is a critical step in activating a brain state characterized by the soothing/contentment emotion regulation system.[1]

> **Recognizing your goodness is an essential feature of self-compassion.**

2. **To begin the work of building a self-compassion image, consider the following two questions:**

   - *What are your good qualities?* What are the positive aspects of how you relate to family, friends, coworkers, and even strangers? What are the good qualities in how you deal with work, daily tasks, and fulfilling civic responsibilities to your community and country? What are some of the positive ways you care for yourself?

   - *Can you think of a person from your past or present, or a spiritual figure like Buddha, Jesus, or Mohammed, or some mythical creation of your own mind, who exhibits ideal compassion?* This person or figure would possess wisdom, inner strength, warmth, love, and nonjudgment. Now imagine how this highly compassionate, caring person would express loving kindness toward you. What might the person notice in you that is good? How would he/she respond to your pain, difficulties, and shortcomings?

3. **Find a quiet place where you can spend some time working on your self-compassion image.** To guide your efforts, you can use the partial Self-Compassion Image Form below as a model, or download the complete form from *www. guilford.com/clark7-forms*. If you find it exceedingly difficult to list your good qualities or to describe a compassionate person, you could consult with a family member, a close friend, or your therapist to help you discover the attributes of self-compassion.

In filling out the Self-Compassion Image Form (see the facing page), Dennis recalled a paternal uncle who treated him with exceptional kindness and understanding as his ideal compassionate other. In the left column he listed personal qualities signifying a capacity for goodness in himself, and in the right column he listed the good qualities of his uncle that were expressions of loving kindness and compassion.

4. **Now start to practice compassionate imaging. Most compassion-focused therapists believe that this is best achieved through mindful meditation. Set aside 15–20 minutes for mindful meditation, and follow these steps.**

TOOL FINDER   Repair Strategy 31 in Chapter 7 describes mindful meditation in full.

Begin by bringing your attention to the breath, paying attention to the soothing rhythm of breathing in and out. Be aware of the rise and fall of your abdomen as you inhale and exhale. Take a couple of minutes to focus on your rhythmic breathing, and then gently shift your attention to the feeling of relaxation in

Self–Compassion Image Form

List of personal goodness (e.g., positive attributes, characteristics)	Qualities of compassionate ideal person
1.	1.
2.	2.

Self-Compassion Image Form: Dennis

List of personal goodness (e.g., positive attributes, characteristics)	Qualities of compassionate ideal person
1. I'm dependable; I always fulfilled my responsibilities and duties in the Army.	1. He would have a deep understanding of human nature—why I feel and behave the way I do.
2. I have courage; I never run away from danger.	2. He would express warmth toward me; he would listen, be patient, and not be quick to give advice.
3. I'm polite and courteous toward others.	3. He would pay attention to me—express concern by looking at me, nodding, and showing that he understands how I feel.
4. I'm patriotic; I love my country and served it well.	4. He would have a soft, quiet, calming voice.
5. I'm honest; I try to be genuine and truthful with people.	5. He would not judge me for being weak or failing, but rather would lovingly accept these faults, knowing that I am fully aware of them myself.
6. I'm loyal to my family and friends; I always watch their backs.	6. He would show strength of conviction, clearly knowing right from wrong.
7. I'm conscientious in my work; I try to do my best.	7. I envision him as a large man with outstretched "bear-like" hands; his eyes have penetrating warmth, and he has a focused, concerned look on his face.
8. I have the potential to take care of my health; in the past, I was always physically fit and careful with my diet.	8. He would frequently acknowledge the pain, the distress that I feel in the moment.
9. I'm a disciplined person, but more so in the past.	9. He would accept the painful memories I bring from the past, and how paralyzed I now feel in the present, because he too has experienced suffering; he knows what it is like to witness unspeakable acts of cruelty.
10. I have a strong sense of moral values.	10. He sees me as having sometimes acted badly, but knows that I am not a bad person.

various parts of your body (the soles of your feet, your shoulders, the back of your neck, etc.). Take 3 minutes or so to attend fully to your body and how it feels to be calm and at peace at this moment in time.

- As you continue in this relaxed, meditative state, shift your attention to the compassionate ideal you've just described. Become that person in your imagination. Adopt that person's posture, facial expression, and tone of voice.

- As you focus your imagination on compassionate wisdom, strength, and nonjudgmental understanding, apply the image to some of the attributes of personal goodness you've previously listed. Imagine you are telling your compassionate person about times when you expressed each of these positive attributes, and feel the warmth, acceptance, and encouragement radiating from your compassionate listener. Spend several minutes imagining this conversation with the compassionate ideal about your goodness.

- Every so often, shift your attention back to your body, back to your breath, and feel the sense of calm and peace associated with meditation. Shift between focused meditation and your compassionate image of goodness several times over a 10- to 15-minute interval before ending your imagery session.

- Finish the imaging practice by bringing your attention back to your body and then your physical surroundings, such as the sounds in the room and then of a more distant part of the house.

5. **You should practice this meditative self-compassion imagery exercise several times a week.** Eventually you will learn to bring the self-compassion image to mind during times when you feel distressed or depressed, and then to use the image to repair your negative mood state. When Dennis felt upset and discouraged with himself for getting stressed out and impatient at work, he could bring to mind his compassionate image. He would imagine his uncle saying to him, "Dennis, you are a good man, reliable, honest, and full of integrity. Your coworkers know they can rely on you when they are in need. You are making progress on patience and letting go of control, but it will take time. Give yourself a chance to break a lifetime habit."

⟩⟩⟩⟩➡ Repair Strategy ㊾: Lovingly Embrace Your Distress

If your mood plummets frequently, distressing events are undoubtedly occurring in your life. Possibly you are struggling with feelings of hurt, rejection, disappointment, or failure. Why not respond to this distress with the self-compassion image developed in the preceding exercise?

Use Repair Strategy 49 when . . .

- you've used Repair Strategy 48 to construct a compassionate ideal. To be truly effective in repairing sad mood, Repair Strategies 48 and 49 should be practiced together.

- you're being especially self-critical and blaming because of mistakes, disappointments, and failures in your life.

- you have a lot of regrets and feel stuck in the past.

REPAIR STRATEGY 49 INSTRUCTIONS

1. **Find a quiet place where you can spend 15–20 minutes in meditation. Take the first 5 minutes to relax and mindfully focus on your breathing.** Alternate this with body scanning, which involves shifting your attention to various parts of the body (your feet, thighs, chest, back, etc.) while focusing on sensations of calm and relaxation in each body region.

> **TOOL FINDER** Details on the mindful breathing and the body scan approaches to meditation are provided in Chapter 7 (Repair Strategy 31).

2. **Once you feel physically calm and at peace with yourself, use your imagination to bring to your mind's eye the compassionate ideal.** Become that person of warmth, acceptance, understanding, and wisdom. Adopt the posture and facial expression of your self-compassionate ideal. Hold that experience of inner strength and nonjudgmental acceptance for several minutes, fully immersed in your imagined self-compassion.

3. **Now bring to your mind the distress, upset, or disappointment you have been feeling.** You can do this by remembering the situation or experience that caused your distress, or by bringing to your mind the person who caused your distress or whom you are now missing in your life. You might even imagine the distress in a more abstract way, giving it the appearance of a dark mythical figure or a black cloud. Whatever your approach, focus your attention on the imagined distress.

4. **Now imagine your self-compassionate ideal responding to this distress, looking at it, and accepting it in a warm, nonjudgmental manner.**

5. **After a couple of minutes, shift back to your body, to the rhythm of your breathing, and reestablish the physical sense of peace and calm. Stay there for a cou-**

ple of minutes, and then go back to the distress image and imagine your compassionate ideal just taking that distress in an embrace—holding it in a loving and accepting manner. The compassionate self does not give advice, nor does it try to solve or eliminate the distress. Rather, this self acknowledges your distress and accepts it for what it is at that moment.

6. **Repeat this alternating shift of attention back and forth between the rhythm of your breathing and the loving embrace of distress for the next 10–15 minutes.**

7. **Make sure you conclude your meditative session with a focus on the breath and feelings of peace and calm.**

Janet found it very easy to bring to her mind the incredible sense of loss and abandonment she had felt when her fiancé broke off their engagement. She could clearly picture the evening he came to her apartment, the shock she felt when he questioned his love for her, and the agony of giving him back the engagement ring. Worst of all, she recalled the intense loneliness and emptiness she felt after he left, as she sat alone in the apartment and wept uncontrollably over the loss of her future. Bringing compassion to that image proved a real challenge.

Janet imagined her grandmother—the "other" whom she had previously used to build her compassionate ideal image. She imagined her grandmother sitting beside this weeping, broken young woman, holding her, stroking her hair, radiating warmth, love, and understanding. She was not talking or giving advice; rather, the compassionate grandmother sat quietly listening, sobbing with her, participating with Janet in her distress. Janet worked with this image, using it repeatedly when she practiced daily self-compassion meditation. Over time Janet found that she was feeling less and less distressed when she recalled the breakup, and that a higher level of acceptance was replacing denial and struggle with this great loss. These feelings were replaced by a realization that her life was moving on and that this moment was different from the past. She was even beginning to see new possibilities as her self-compassion enveloped this great hurt from the past.

⫸➡ Repair Strategy ㊿: Do unto Others

Have you ever met a kind person you didn't like? Now contrast this kind person with a self-centered person who thinks only of him-/herself, or, even worse, a stingy or miserly person. Don't you find these people much harder to like? Don't you really want to avoid them, because they generate negative feelings, conflict, and resentment? The fact is, we all are drawn to people who express kindness to others. And kindness

is good for our mental health; it benefits both the givers and the receivers. If you show kindness to others, they are more likely to be kind to you; they will be drawn to you and show appreciation, and you'll feel good about yourself.[1]

From the smallest gestures of kindness (such as a smile, opening the door, or letting others go first) to larger acts (such as giving gifts, spending time with someone in need or suffering, or volunteering), acts of kindness can be contagious in their positive effects on self and others. In a recent Japanese study of university students,[3] happy people were kinder and became even happier and more grateful when asked to record their acts of kindness for 1 week. We can assume that simply keeping track of their acts of kindness probably increased the amount of kindness they showed to others. So kindness improves mood state, which means that it can be a powerful source of mood repair for self and others.

I was reminded of the good feeling that kindness brings just a couple of days ago. My wife and I decided it was time for lunch, and so we approached the hostess at a popular, very busy restaurant. The place was crowded, and the hostess said the wait would be at least 40 minutes. As we were deciding whether to stay or not, a total stranger approached me and offered his buzzer, saying that he and his wife had decided not to stay. He thought they had only about 10 minutes left on their buzzer, but I had to remember to listen for the name "John" to be called. We shook hands, and I thanked him for his kindness. Sure enough, within a few minutes John's name was called, and our wait time was cut short. But what is interesting is that for the next 10 minutes or so, I had such a positive, good feeling as I thought about John's small act of kindness. I wonder whether John was also feeling good about sharing his buzzer, or whether maybe he just got on with his shopping.

Researchers are just beginning to understand the positive effects of kindness and generosity toward others. Even a tiny act of kindness, like smiling at a person, can have a positive impact. The smile will be interpreted as an expression of happiness, which is then contagious, so the person receiving the happy emotion will mimic the happiness and even show a positive attitude shift (especially if the receiver likes the happy person). There is evidence that genuine smiling can reduce the effects of negative affect and is associated with better emotional adjustment.[4] More obvious examples of kindness, such as witnessing acts of generosity or virtue, can make us feel lifted up or inspired; this can lead to a more compassionate view of others and can lower daily depressed mood, even in people struggling with clinical depression or anxiety. In one study, individuals with clinical depression or anxiety completed daily ratings of feeling competent, morally uplifted, and compassionate toward others, as well as the extent of felt emotional closeness and kindness from others, over a 10-day period. The researchers found that participants felt less depressed and hostile on days when they rated themselves higher in compassion and receiving closeness and kindness from others.[5]

Thus there is a very tight link between kindness and generosity on the one hand and positive emotion on the other. Having more kindness and generosity in your life is a powerful strategy for lifting yourself out of the doldrums of a depressed mood. Acts of kindness toward others may not come naturally to you, or you may not feel like extending yourself to others because of low mood—but if you become intentional and try out small acts of kindness, you can begin to experience their positive effects in your life.

Use Repair Strategy 50 if you . . .

- struggle with a negative and cynical outlook on life more generally.
- have difficulty trusting other people.
- feel hurt, rejected, or abandoned.
- tend to be aloof or distant from others.
- have been quite self-focused—preoccupied with your own problems and negative emotional state.

REPAIR STRATEGY 50 INSTRUCTIONS

So what can you do to build more kindness in your daily life? The following are some steps you can take to inject more generosity and virtue into your daily life.

1. **Recognize kindness.** It is likely that acts of kindness are happening all around you but go unnoticed. Increase your awareness of kindness. Do you know any kind people in your life? If so, how do they exhibit kindness and generosity to others? When you are around these people, what do you observe in how they interact with others? Do they smile? Do they show interest in other people's lives? Are they quick to help out? You might even want to make a kindness or generosity list to help you recognize common acts of kindness.

2. **Focus on close friends or family members.** Select two or three people in your life who are close to you, such as a spouse/partner, parent, child, or close friend. What could you do that would involve acts of kindness toward them? Plan on doing some of these things, and then notice the impact on the person receiving your kindness, as well as on your own feelings.

3. **Increase behaviors that will make others want to interact with you.** There are a number of communication skills you can use to increase people's desire to interact with you. For example, showing that you are interested and care about what is happening in the lives of your coworkers and friends is a powerful incentive for others to be around you. Asking people about their day or about some difficulty in

their lives, and expressing recognition of their accomplishments or of good things that happen to them, are other examples of positive social gestures. One of your goals could be to have a brief conversation each day with a friend or coworker in which you ask about the person's life, practicing a mindfully compassionate approach as you listen to what he/she is telling you.

4. **Perform random acts of kindness.** Every day we interact with dozens of people— at work, in stores, on the street, even in traffic. How often do you express "random acts of kindness"? Do you let in a driver who is trying to switch lanes? Do you offer your seat on the subway to a person who is carrying a lot of parcels or who looks exceptionally tired? Do you hold the door open for people, or let someone who has a couple of tired and restless children go ahead of you in line? Do you show patience, kindness, and appreciation to clerks, waiters, or even call center employees who are trying to serve you? All of these situations involve minor acts or gestures of kindness that can set the tone for your day and influence your mood state.

5. **Consider volunteerism.** Do you engage in any volunteer work in your community? Volunteerism is an excellent way to express kindness and generosity on a larger scale. Volunteering opens up opportunities to interact with others, but it can also be very uplifting as you contribute in a positive way to a much bigger community initiative. At the beginning of this chapter, I have mentioned a friend who found her volunteer work at a soup kitchen important in coping with the distress of cancer treatment. If you are not doing some volunteer work, consider how you might make room for this activity, even on a limited basis.

Stoking the Fires of Compassion

As you conclude this chapter, you may be thinking that what I have recommended here is all common sense. After all, the take-home message could be boiled down to "Be kind and forgiving to yourself and others. If you do these things, you'll feel a lot less depressed and more positive about life." But don't be fooled by the simplicity of the message. Practicing kindness and compassion to yourself and to others can be very hard to do, especially when you're feeling down. It starts by being intentional about seeing the goodness, love, and caring in yourself and other people.

Science is backing up what we might know from common sense—that self-compassion and kindness toward others have positive effects on emotional health and well-being. Researchers have consistently found that individuals who experience more compassion have lower levels of depression, anxiety, and stress. In a series of studies conducted at Duke University, researchers found that students who reported more self-compassion in response to daily negative events had less negative emotion, had lower negative feelings about themselves, and were calmer in how they handled negative events. In the same study, highly self-compassionate students were less likely to ruminate or have self-critical thoughts when faced with failure, and were less reactive to both positive and negative feedback.[6]

As you begin each day, look for opportunities to express tolerance, understanding, and empathy toward your own pain and difficulties, as well as those of others. An intentional focus on compassion and loving kindness can be a powerful mood repair strategy. However, you will probably find compassion-focused mood repair most successful when combined with the other repair strategies discussed in this book.

TOOL FINDER

- If your attempts at self-compassion are blocked by highly self-critical thoughts and beliefs, consult the cognitive mood repair strategies in Chapter 4.
- If you have trouble taking a gentler, more positive approach to yourself, practice doing some of the more concrete pleasure and enjoyment activities in Chapter 5.
- If you are having difficulty with compassion-focused meditation (Repair Strategy 48), go back to mindfulness meditation as described in Chapter 7.
- If you are not achieving mood benefits with the compassion-focused strategies, you may need to combine these strategies with work on positive mood and gratitude as discussed in Chapter 14.

12 get active, stay fit, and be well

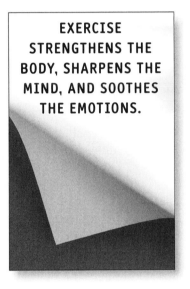

EXERCISE STRENGTHENS THE BODY, SHARPENS THE MIND, AND SOOTHES THE EMOTIONS.

Being healthy is a real challenge in the 21st century. Most of us spend long hours sitting inactive in front of screens at home and work; consuming highly processed foods for meals and snacks; and getting minimal sleep because of our highly demanding, stressful lives. For years, health researchers have warned about the ill effects of such a lifestyle on our overall health. Now there is solid scientific evidence that physical inactivity, poor diet, and lack of sleep have adverse effects on our emotional well-being, too. In fact, we now know that physical exercise, better diet, and regular sleep can improve our mood states. So we must include self-care practices in any effective approach to mood repair. Of course, this is easier said than done. We have all tried to change our lifestyle at one time or another, and doing this feels like the hardest thing ever. It seems as if every aspect of modern life conspires against healthy living. This is clearly illustrated by Andrea and Mark, who represent two opposing approaches to physical health and well-being.

Andrea was a married mother of three teenagers and a part-time dance instructor. There was intensity, even enthusiasm about her; she was a highly artistic and talented person who in every way was fully engaged in life. But despite the appearance that she was leading the good life, the blues had stalked Andrea for many years. After trying different treatment approaches, Andrea decided that what she needed was an overhaul in her lifestyle. So she started taking more care with her diet, established a more regular sleep routine, and took up running. Of course, Andrea approached these lifestyle changes as she did everything else—with an unsurpassable intensity and determination. She built up her endurance and eventually decided to train for a marathon. She ran her first marathon 5 years ago, and after that ran a race or two every year. Andrea claimed that running, eating well, and getting enough sleep transformed her battle with depression. No longer did she experience long periods of feeling down and depressed. She couldn't believe how much better she felt mentally and emotionally as a result of her newfound enthusiasm for running.

Mark, a 44-year-old manager of a real estate office, described feeling down, gloomy, and pessimistic more days than not. He attributed much of his struggle with low mood to the downturn in the economy, especially its effects on the real estate market. He had had to lay off employees and had seen his own income plummet. At one time Mark had been physically fit. In his 20s he was a regular fixture at the gym, lifting weights, doing cardio training, and being careful with his diet. He admitted that back then he'd felt great—positive, energetic, and full of optimism. But in the last 10 years he'd given up on exercise. His diet centered on fast food, which felt like an evil necessity due to his work schedule. He had trouble sleeping, started smoking, and drank more than he should. Mark noted that he had tried to change his lifestyle, but each time he "fell off the wagon" within a few weeks. He knew what he should do but couldn't seem to do it, and so he ended up stuck in the blues, disgusted with his lack of discipline and determination. He had also gained weight, and his doctor started warning him that he was putting his health at risk.

Mark and Andrea obviously represent opposing attitudes toward physical self-care. Andrea developed a passion for running that became a powerful mood repair strategy in her life, whereas Mark struggled to make lifestyle changes, even though he knew they would improve his mental and physical health. Most of us probably fall somewhere in the middle when it comes to taking care of our health. Although good physical self-care is an important contributor to positive mood, we struggle to get started or maintain healthy behavioral practices. Since staying motivated is the number one challenge to healthy living, in this chapter I focus primarily on ways you can strengthen your motivation and resolve to practice healthy behavior.

This chapter also places a particular emphasis on physical exercise. The scientific evidence for direct mood repair benefits is strongest for exercise. You may feel more motivated, once you know how clearly the research demonstrates that regular physical exercise can immediately improve negative mood and even reduce the risk of depression.

Why Care?: The Benefits of Regular Exercise

The road to better physical health is paved with good intentions but littered with poor retention. Even though most people recognize the importance of physical fitness, the vast majority of individuals who start an exercise program fail to follow through. Some begin and then give up after a few days or weeks. There are even dedicated exercisers who stop suddenly after years of maintaining a regular exercise schedule. One of my friends ran several times a week for 25 years, and then suddenly stopped running after experiencing a health issue that did not require cessation of his running. I have been running for 15 years, and yet I still go through periods when I struggle with my motivation to exercise.

In their book *Exercise for Mood and Anxiety,* Michael Otto and Jasper Smits contend that we struggle with motivation because we exercise for the wrong reasons.[1] If we focus on the mood-improving qualities of exercise, we're more likely to stay motivated—*because the mood-elevating effects of exercise can be felt immediately, after a single exercise session.* If, on the other hand, we exercise to lose weight or improve our physical appearance, we're more likely to get discouraged and quit, because it takes so long to see results in those areas.

> **To stick with exercise, focus on its immediate mood-healing effects.**

So if you begin exercising to feel better, you have a better chance of sticking with it. Of course, actually getting out, being active, and feeling better will be the best way to motivate yourself to stick with it. Another way to bolster your resolve to exercise is to be more aware of the scientific basis for exercise—to hear about its documented effects on your health and well-being. Having accurate health information is an important part of staying healthy and fit. See the sidebar "Exercise as a Mood Enhancer" on page 206.

Maybe you're already aware of the accumulated research data in favor of exercise, yet you have had trouble starting an exercise program in the past. Knowing why might increase your chances of success this time around.

⫸⫸ Repair Strategy 51: Consult the Exercise Motivation Checklist

Use the following checklist to identify your motivation "weak spots," and then be on the lookout for these problems when you renew your exercise program.

- ❑ *Aversion to pain*: Strenuous exercise requires considerable effort, and pushing your body to its limits can feel very unpleasant. Consider your tolerance level for physical discomfort. Will you need to improve your pain tolerance to break through that initial period of high physical discomfort?

- ❑ *Misguided goals*: Did you start exercising to lose weight or achieve a more sculpted body, only to give up because you were not getting the results you expected?

exercise as a mood enhancer

There is compelling scientific evidence that moderate- to high-intensity physical exercise is a powerful mood repair strategy. For example, in a review of 70 intervention studies, Vicki Conn at the University of Missouri found that physical activity, whether supervised by a researcher or done at home, significantly reduced depressive symptoms in otherwise healthy people without clinical depression.[2] Moreover, low-intensity supervised interventions involving a combined focus on endurance (e.g., running), flexibility (e.g., stretching), and resistance (e.g., weight lifting) were more effective than a single focus on endurance, such as only running on your own at home. It turns out that regular exercise is also as effective as antidepressant medication in treating clinical depression, and individuals taking antidepressants may find that the addition of an exercise regimen boosts the effects of medication.[3] Physical exercise also reduces stress, decreases negative thinking and rumination, enhances positive mood and cognitive functioning, and actually increases longevity.

Not surprisingly, being sedentary has negative effects on emotional health. A recent Brazilian study found that people who reported engaging in physical activity twice a week or less were twice as likely to report depressive or anxious symptoms than people who said they were physically active three or more times a week.[4]

Recently I did a 10-km run in 57 minutes and burned 760 calories. Later in the day I ate a piece of my favorite cheesecake, only to discover that it contained over 800 calories. So 10 minutes of eating equaled the calorie-reducing impact of almost 1 hour of continuous high-intensity running! Exercise should be part of any weight reduction program, but the effect of exercise on weight loss is minimal. Exercising to feel good and improve your cognitive ability is a goal that can be realized much more quickly; knowing this can boost your motivation and commitment.

❑ *Giving in to procrastination:* This issue is Public Enemy Number 1 for any exercise program, and probably everyone could check this one off as a motivation killer. We all battle the temptation to procrastinate, and if you've given up on exercise in the past, it's likely that procrastination played a big part. At this moment I am battling procrastination. It's early morning, and I've arisen to work on this chapter. I've been given a tight deadline, and so I'm feeling under the gun. I'm making great progress, but as the time ticks by, I realize I should stop working and do my early morning run. I think about postponing the run until after work. I convince myself that I'm making important progress in the writing and shouldn't interrupt the flow. Besides, it's cold and dark outside, and I don't feel like running now. So am I procrastinating, or am I being practical and flexible? Of course, time will tell. If I actually do my run after work, I'm being flexible. If I don't get the run in, then I've fallen prey to procrastination. (Postscript: I didn't get the run in, but I did go the following day!) Delaying your exercise at any given moment is not the problem; it's a pattern of continued delay that undermines motivation. The strategies presented below are designed to help you avoid a pattern of procrastination.

> **TOOL FINDER** If you have problems with procrastination more generally, and not just with exercise, you'll want to spend time with the mood repair strategies in Chapter 13.

- *Short-sightedness:* This problem goes hand in hand with procrastination. We can easily become short-sighted; that is, we can convince ourselves to put off exercise until the future, because we'll have more time then.[1] But we tend to underestimate all the demands that will be placed on us in the future, which means that in reality the best time to do your exercise is now, not later. You might think, "I'll go to the gym after work, when I'll have more time," but of course you fail to acknowledge that you often stay at work late and you promised to drive the kids to their sports events when you got home. You won't have more time after work; in fact, you'll probably have less. And so another day goes by without exercise.

- *Slippage effects:* Anyone who has tried to change a lifestyle behavior like diet, exercise, smoking, or drinking will experience setbacks. No one can maintain a perfect exercise schedule all the time. Unfortunately, we are usually most vulnerable to quitting during setbacks. I am amazed at how hard it is to start exercising again if I've taken time off due to sickness, injury, or travel. Of course the minute I start again, I recognize its benefits, but that doesn't help beforehand! Dealing with setbacks or slack periods in your exercise program is an important part of staying motivated.

- *"Busyitis":* OK, I made up this term, but how many times have you heard people say (or have you said to yourself), "I don't have the time; my life is too busy"? Of course you have a busy and demanding life, and it always will be that way. The fact is, however, we make room for the things that are important to us. People who exercise regularly are not less busy and productive than sedentary

> **Making time to feel better, work better, and prolong your life has big payoffs.**

individuals are. In fact some of the busiest, most productive, and most successful people I've met engage in regular exercise. I believe you will experience the benefits of physical exercise and realize it's worth the investment in time. Recently I asked a young woman who is a mother, a busy academic, and a productive researcher how she found the time for her ambitious exercise program. She explained that she viewed it as "me time"—a time when she indulged herself and recharged her batteries so she could pursue her demanding life.

Getting Started

Now that you've identified the challenges to your motivation, it's time to get started with exercise. Throughout, it's important to keep your focus on why you are exercising: *to experience the good feeling that arises when you finish your physical activity.*

Use the fitness approach to mood repair if you . . .

- are overweight and physically unfit.
- have a sedentary lifestyle.
- feel highly stressed and overwhelmed.
- experience low energy and fatigue.
- have trouble concentrating and making decisions.
- have sleep difficulties.

The hardest part of any exercise program is getting started (or restarting after a long period of no exercise). The following strategies highlight some of the most important steps to get you going.

▶▶▶▶ Repair Strategy 52: Choose the Right Physical Activity

REPAIR STRATEGY 52 INSTRUCTIONS

1. **Have a physical checkup, and tell your family doctor that you intend to start exercising.** This is especially important if you are over 40 years old, are overweight, and/or have health issues (a personal or family history of cardiovascular disease, diabetes, high blood pressure, etc.). Take the advice of your family doctor

seriously, and follow the doctor's recommendations on the nature and intensity of your exercise program.

2. **Select aerobic, anaerobic, or some combination of physical activity.** Aerobic activity is exercise that increases your need for oxygen and accelerates your heart rate (brisk walking, running, cycling, swimming, rowing, dancing, etc.). Anaerobic exercise, such as weight lifting or sprinting, involves strengthening major muscle groups and can also be effective in reducing depression. If you choose mainly anaerobic exercise, include at least some aerobic activity, since some studies suggest that aerobic activity may have a slight edge in mood improvement. Also, get at least a moderate level of exercise. Exercise durations of at least 10 minutes are recommended to achieve mood improvement.[1] One of the great benefits of more vigorous exercise is that it interferes with the normal thinking process, so that it becomes more difficult to worry and ruminate, although your workout may need to last 20 minutes or more before rumination starts to fade.[1] If you can talk but not sing during exercise, intensity is moderate; being able to speak only a few words before catching your breath is high-intensity; panting and being unable to talk at all mean you're pushing yourself too hard and should slow down.

> **Choose a moderate-intensity aerobic activity for the best mood enhancement effects.**

The World Health Organization and the U.S. Department of Health and Human Services recommend at least 2.5 hours per week of moderate-intensity aerobic physical activity for periods of 10 minutes or longer, or at least 1.25 hours per week of high-intensity aerobic physical exercise or some equivalent combination of moderate- and vigorous-intensity activity.[5, 6] Here are some examples of moderate-intensity exercise:

- Walking at 3–4 mph
- Bicycling on flat ground at 10–12 mph
- Leisurely swimming

Here are some examples of high-intensity exercise:

- Running at more than 4.5 mph
- Bicycling on flat ground at more than 12 mph
- Cross-country skiing at more than 2.5 mph

Whatever your exercise activity, you should be sweating, breathing more rapidly, and elevating your heart rate, although your target should be 60–85% of your maximum heart rate.

3. **Select a physical activity that gives you some enjoyment.** The higher your pleasure during or after exercise, the more likely you'll be to keep it up.

4. **Consider hiring a fitness trainer.** If you've never really exercised or you've had several years of sedentary living, consulting an expert is wise. Practically every gym has trainers available to advise members for a fee. A consultant or trainer will assess your current level of fitness, start you at an appropriate level of physical activity, provide a graduated program of exercise, and offer repeated assessments of your progress. Meeting with a fitness expert also provides a source of accountability that will help with motivation.

⟫⟫→ Repair Strategy ⑬: Take It Slow

REPAIR STRATEGY 53 INSTRUCTIONS

1. **Determine your baseline fitness level.** Your age, weight, physical health, and daily activity level will determine your baseline fitness level. If you expect too much and push yourself too hard at the beginning, pain and discomfort will urge you to quit. This is another area in which a trainer can help, and possibly some advice from your family physician may be useful as well. (See Repair Strategy 52, just above.)

2. **Make sure you have the proper clothing, footwear, and other equipment.** It's important to feel as comfortable as possible while working out, so you don't give yourself another reason to give up. You will be amazed at how quickly you heat up, so make sure your clothing is cool and can deal with excessive sweating. The proper footwear is essential to reduce risk of injury.

3. **Consider joining a gym or an exercise group.** Joining a fitness class—an aerobics class at the gym or a running clinic sponsored by your local running equipment retail store, for example—is a great way to get started, because the program will be structured and scheduled at regular times. Paying for classes and participating in a group are great ways to increase accountability, which helps instill commitment to regular physical exercise. If classes are not for you, try to do your running, walking, or cycling with a friend or group of fellow workout enthusiasts. Exercising with others increases interest and enjoyment and again creates accountability. For years I did early-morning runs with a group of men, and many times I would force myself out of bed to avoid letting my friends down.

⋙➡ Repair Strategy ㊻: Plan Your Workout

REPAIR STRATEGY 54 INSTRUCTIONS

1. **Choose the best time of the day to do your physical exercise.** What time of day works best for you to exercise—early morning, lunchtime, after work? Whatever you choose, stick to your schedule. Varying it will increase procrastination and missed exercise sessions. You should give yourself 2–3 rest days a week, so that your body has a chance to recover.

2. **Establish a workout routine.** Tasks that are routine take less effort to initiate from day to day. Once exercise becomes a routine part of your day, you'll find yourself just doing it, almost without thought.

3. **Vary your workout.** Routine is important, but you do want to inject some variety into your workout to maintain interest and enjoyment. Avoid doing the same thing day after day after day. For example, if you are running, vary your route, the distance, and whether you run alone or with a friend. Often runners will do a longer run on the weekend and shorter runs during the week. Doing both aerobic and anaerobic activities will also keep things varied.

4. **Start an exercise log.** The next section of this chapter, on staying motivated, introduces a Weekly Exercise Log that can be used to keep track of your workouts. It's a good idea to start the log at the beginning of your exercise program, so you have a record of your progress from the first day onward. This can be a great incentive and source of motivation as you look back on how little physical activity you could do when you started. This is especially true for aerobic activities like running, cycling, and swimming, where you can easily see the longer times and distances you are now able to achieve with regular exercise.

Staying Motivated

You need to take your exercise program one day at a time. No matter how long you've been engaged in a regular exercise routine, your day-to-day motivation will waver. Some days you'll finish on a real high, feeling especially rejuvenated and invigorated after your routine; on other days, sticking to your commitment will feel like a real struggle, and you'll leave your workout session with nothing but relief that it's over. That's why the strategies for staying motivated often focus on heightening awareness of the benefits you've gotten—even when they seem small in proportion to your effort on that particular day.

it's not too late to start exercising

Maybe you've read to this point but are thinking to yourself, "I can't do this; it's too late for me to start exercising." For the vast majority of people, it is never too late. My wife, who at this writing is 55 years old, started regular exercise 9 months ago, having never participated in sports or regular exercise in her youth or middle adult years. I've asked her to share her experience with taking up running in her own words.

"I have never been a fan of sweating. I did not participate in organized sports when I was young—in fact, I even tried on occasion to get excused from gym class as a teenager. And, though I have always been an active person engaged with life through a variety of activities, you would never mistake me for an athlete. Give me gardening, or an afternoon of recreational skiing. But, please, never call on me when you want someone to go work out with you.

"Well, all that changed, or started to change, last January. Like many women over 50, I was 25 pounds heavier now than when I got pregnant for the first time. With our nest empty, and a 4-month sabbatical in Florida to work on our next books, I decided that this might be the moment to face the inevitable—I needed to exercise for the sake of my own health.

"I always had plenty of excuses as to why it was not possible for me to engage in regular exercise—including our children and their schedules, my own demanding professional responsibilities, work travel, David's chaotic schedule, my own volunteer activities, and on the list went. Besides, I did not even know if I was physically able to begin and sustain a rigorous physical exercise program.

"At first I kept my newfound determination about exercise a secret. I started to walk early in the mornings when David would go for his 5- or 6-mile run. At the end of week 2, I decided to try jogging a bit—I would run between two telephone poles along our route, or I would choose a tree several hundred yards away and run as far as there. It was exceptionally hard. I was out of breath. I hated it. But I persevered. In a few more weeks, I had worked up to a run/walk pattern until I was running about 60% and walking 40%. It was now 6 weeks into my routine, and it was clear to me that I was making some modest gains, like I was no longer gasping after running 100 yards!

"Our two 20-something daughters came to visit us in Florida for their end-of-February breaks from their respective universities. When one daughter ran with her father, the other one went walking and running with me. They were so pleased with my progress and pushed me to go farther and faster. My ability to do this surprised even me. When they left, I was determined to see what I could do left to my own devices. That was the first time that I completed the 7 kilometers of running on my own."

➤➤➤ Repair Strategy 55: Monitor Your Progress

The Weekly Exercise Log on the next page is an example of a form that can keep you motivated by providing instant feedback. Feel free to make copies, or print them out from *www.guilford.com/clark7-forms*.

REPAIR STRATEGY 55 INSTRUCTIONS

1. **Maintain an accurate record.** Complete your log immediately after each workout, so that your entries are clear and accurate. If you wait to complete the log later, your observations about the effects of exercise on mood may be distorted by intervening events.

2. **When you fill out your log, ask yourself whether it generally seems to be taking less effort to engage in exercise.** Are you noticing an increase in enjoyment during your workouts? How are your workouts affecting your mood later in the day? Keeping the Weekly Exercise Log will help you stay focused on improved mood as the goal for physical exercise; it will also curb procrastination and nip slippage in the bud.

3. **Review the log periodically.** It's important to take particular notice of increases over time in duration, intensity, and distance. This provides you with objective data on improved physical fitness. You might even want to write a summary that states how far you've come in your fitness level (e.g., "I could only run 15 minutes for 1.5 miles, but now I run 30 minutes and can do 3 miles. Imagine me running 3 miles!"). You can use these as "fitness statements" to motivate yourself to keep going.

4. **Review the log for mood effects.** Take particular notice of what you've recorded in the last column of the log. Are you seeing higher enjoyment ratings the longer you exercise? Is there evidence that exercise is having an immediate positive effect on your mood? Documented evidence that you are feeling better can be a greater motivator.

➤➤➤ Repair Strategy 56: Maintain Your Exercise Routine

There are different things you can do to make exercise a habit. For example, have your workout clothes prepared and set your alarm if you choose to exercise in the early morning. If you have trouble getting up or out the door to the gym, focus on one step at a time, and tell yourself you'll do a light workout today. Pair the workout with some-

Weekly Exercise Log

Name: _____ Date from: _____ to: _____

Instructions: Complete the log after each exercise session. Periodically review your weekly logs to evaluate your physical fitness progress.

Day	Exercise activity	Duration	Effort (0–10)	Enjoy-ment (0–10)	Observed effects on mood state during and after exercise
Mon.					
Tues.					
Weds.					
Thurs.					
Fri.					
Sat.					
Sun.					

Note. Duration: Length of exercise session (minutes). Effort: Rate degree of effort needed to complete the exercise, from 0 (exercised with ease) to 10 (exceedingly difficult; took everything in my power to finish the exercise session). Enjoyment: Rate degree of enjoyment during and immediately after the exercise session, from 0 (not even a moment of enjoyment) to 10 (almost continuous enjoyment during and after exercise). Observed effects: What were you thinking and feeling during your exercise session and afterwards? Were there any noticeable effects on negative mood, depressive rumination, worry, or self-criticism?

thing enjoyable that you don't do on rest days. Remind your spouse/partner or your exercise buddy that you'll be out tomorrow for the workout. Creating repetition will make exercise a routine activity that will turn it into a more automatic, less effortful habit.

⤏⤏⤏➡ Repair Strategy 57: Diversify Your Exercise Routine

Pursuing a mixture of exercise activities will increase your enjoyment, which in turn will encourage persistence with your exercise program.

REPAIR STRATEGY 57 INSTRUCTIONS

1. **As suggested earlier in the chapter, alternate between aerobic and anaerobic exercise.** You'll get the increased benefit of both kinds of exercise, while also sustaining your interest and motivation.

2. **Consult a trainer about a combination of exercises you're considering, to ensure getting a moderately intense workout that improves mood.**

3. **If you can't come up with ideas for varying your routine on your own, consult any of the many excellent websites that offer advice and workout plans (e.g.,** *www.crossfit.com, www.fitness.com, www.fitness.gov,* **etc.).** Most of these are free, but may require that you register to get access to their resources.

4. **Be prepared that initially new activities may feel difficult to integrate into your routine.** As your workout becomes more habitual, you might be surprised to find that it's hard to introduce another activity, like cycling or swimming. Deviating from your usual routine may make it harder to judge your physical limits, meaning that you may feel more comfortable and confident when doing a familiar workout. Use the other strategies in this chapter to push through this barrier. Also, remind yourself that cross-training may be helpful if you are experiencing considerable pain and discomfort with exercise.

⤏⤏⤏➡ Repair Strategy 58: Capitalize on Accountability

The designers of intervention programs have known for years that we're more likely to maintain behavioral change when we declare our intentions publicly and when others join us in our efforts. This is one of the important elements of diets, for example: Attending group meetings introduces peer accountability, which encourages adherence to the diet regimen. So use accountability to your advantage. It can reduce procrastination and slippage by encouraging adherence to your workout routine. Here are some ways to make yourself accountable.

REPAIR STRATEGY 58 INSTRUCTIONS

1. **Work out with friends or in a group.** This is as important to maintaining your motivation for exercise as it is for getting started.

2. **Share your exercise experiences with interested friends and family members (without being obnoxious).** Over time physical fitness will become part of your identity, and you'll feel an obligation to maintain the image. You'll feel embarrassed to admit that you haven't exercised in a while. So this subtle social pressure or accountability can encourage you to "soldier on" with your daily exercise.

➤ Repair Strategy 59: Think Small

Thinking about spending the next 30–45 minutes in vigorous physical exertion will feel daunting and deplete the energy needed to initiate your exercise activity. I can tell you from experience that thinking about spending the next 50 minutes running 8 or 9 kilometers feels overwhelming and makes me reluctant to get started. So the best strategy is to break down your exercise session into small steps.

REPAIR STRATEGY 59 INSTRUCTIONS

1. **First, think about getting dressed and ready for your exercise session.**

2. **Then get started, telling yourself that you'll go slow and easy.**

3. **As you warm up and start to feel better, you can extend your exercise duration and intensity by focusing on just the next 5 minutes, and so on.** You can keep extending your target duration in this way until you finish the exercise session. The key is to stay focused on the present and not to dwell on the future—that is, on how much time or distance is left in your exercise session.

4. **Limit how often you check the clock.** Clock watching will make the time go much slower and keep you focused on how much time is left in your exercise session. Many people who use a

> Hide clocks and distance gauges on exercise equipment, so you stay focused on the moment while exercising.

treadmill place a towel over the digital time and distance gauges to reduce clock watching.

⏩ Repair Strategy 60: Use Music and Other Diversions

Listening to your favorite music can increase your enjoyment of and persistence with exercise. There are now many types of devices that can deliver music while you exercise. The key is to use music you like and to vary it over time, in order to maintain interest and reduce boredom. Music is also a great distraction from thinking about negative physical sensations, and it has a powerful influence on mood state. In addition, you can watch your favorite television program or read a book if using exercise equipment. The goal is to keep the exercise session interesting and diverse so you don't become overly focused on physical exertion and fatigue. Diana Nyad, the 64-year-old American endurance swimmer who completed a 110-mile swim from Cuba to Key West, Florida, in 2013, commented in a CNN interview that music played an important role in keeping her going, especially during the two nights of swimming. Listening to your favorite music while exercising can also improve pain and discomfort tolerance.

⏩ Repair Strategy 61: Take a Mindful Approach to Exercise

Mindfulness can also be used to increase your motivation to exercise. Specifically, it can enable you to become more aware of the physical sensations and emotions you experience during exercise.[1] This involves acknowledging what you're actually feeling, and accepting your experience in a nonjudgmental fashion without becoming overly consumed by it.

I can't stress enough the importance of adopting a mindful approach that focuses on more positive, pleasant thoughts and sensations, while diverting attention away from negative thinking and unpleasant physical sensations. Over the years I have been amazed at the power of attention while I am running. If I focus on aches, pains, and fatigue, or on my negative thoughts of exhaustion and wanting to quit, it feels as if I am running in Army boots. The amount of effort needed is 10-fold. However, if I shift attention to my surroundings and to pleasant sensations, and take particular notice of feeling strong and more energetic, the effort I need to continue diminishes dramatically.

REPAIR STRATEGY 61 INSTRUCTIONS

1. **Review the mindfulness instructions in Chapter 7 before trying to apply mindfulness to exercise.** Be aware of the focus of your attention. Are you attending to aches, pains, and breathlessness, or to feelings of strength and vitality?

2. **Notice your sensations and feelings during exercise, and react to them in a way that reduces distress through acceptance.** For example, assume that halfway through a run you become aware of terrible fatigue and think, "I can't continue; I'm going to have to stop." A mindful approach to this experience would be to detach yourself from the fatigue and observe it:

   > "Isn't this interesting? All of a sudden I feel exhausted, but it's only in my legs and breathing; I've had this feeling before. Welcome back, fatigue. I'm obviously giving myself a good workout; and that negative thought of not being able to finish, I've seen that thought before. I've not been overwhelmed by it in the past. I can choose to let the fatigue thought pass by and shift my attention to the landscape around me. I've been good at shifting my attention in the past. What I need to do is focus on the moment, and I can certainly go with these feelings and sensations for the next few minutes. I can shift my attention to more pleasant experiences, such as the environment around me, my feelings of strength, and the knowledge that I am actually improving my fitness. That's what I'll do. I've really been learning new skills at coaching myself through fatigue and negative thoughts."

3. **Be attentive to positive feelings, to fuel physical activity and reduce the effort needed to complete your routine.** A mindful perspective can improve tolerance for the pain and discomfort of intense physical exertion.

⫸ Repair Strategy 62: Correct Negative Exercise Self-Talk

Our thoughts have a powerful impact on our motivation to exercise. Nothing erodes motivation faster than self-criticism. Be vigilant for negative thoughts:

"I'm not making any progress."

"Why bother? This isn't helping me get over my depression."

"I'm so slow or awkward; I'm just not cut out to exercise."

"I look so fat and ugly."

"I'll never feel better."

"It's too hard."

"I need my sleep; I'll exercise tomorrow."

"This run really sucked; I may as well give up."

Not only will this type of thinking make you feel more depressed, but you will quickly convince yourself to give up on exercise as a mood repair strategy.

TOOL FINDER   Chapter 4 discusses how negative self-critical thinking intensifies a depressive mood state; it then provides strategies for reducing this kind of thinking.

REPAIR STRATEGY 62 INSTRUCTIONS

1. **First, be aware of your negative thinking before, during, or after exercising.** Of course, you don't want to focus *all* your attention on negative thoughts, but at least catch yourself when your mind begins to turn negative (e.g., "I must look ridiculous; I feel so exhausted; I'm falling behind everyone else in the class").

2. **Use the evidence-gathering format discussed in Chapter 4 to challenge the negative thoughts (see Repair Strategy 12).** Do this in a gentle manner, without getting into an argument with yourself. Ask yourself, "Am I thinking about exercise accurately, or am I being overly negative and self-critical?"

3. **Generate a more accurate, realistic evaluation of your exercise session.** Ask yourself, "What is a more realistic, helpful alternative view on my attempts at getting physically fit and improving my mood?" For example, you might remind yourself that you've made tremendous progress in your physical fitness; that you must expect both good and bad exercise days; and that regardless of how difficult the workout may seem, you will feel better for doing your routine.

4. **Redirect your attention to positive thoughts about exercise, and appreciate the gains you've made since starting to exercise.** You might want to generate a list of more encouraging ways to think about physical exertion during exercise. For example, when I'm beginning to feel fatigue and weakness when running, I turn my attention to my legs, heart, or lungs and think about how well they are working to carry me this distance. I also imagine how they are getting a good workout and

actually becoming stronger with the exercise. I find these positive thoughts a lot more encouraging and inspirational for actually finishing the run.

Sleep

There is a strong connection between sleep deprivation and depression. Sleep difficulties are both signs of and contributors to clinical depression. However, even a few nights with 1–2 hours less sleep can have adverse effects, such as irritability, poor concentration and memory, reduced energy, fatigue, decreased ability to cope with stress, and general malaise. Thus consistent failure to acquire sufficient sleep will contribute to more negative mood—and, obviously, greater difficulty in adhering to a regular exercise program.

It is estimated that 10% of American adults get insufficient sleep each night; that 38% fail to obtain sufficient sleep 7 or more days per month; and that 50–70 million Americans are chronically sleep-deprived. Although the National Sleep Foundation recommends that healthy adults get 7–9 hours of daily sleep, the Centers for Disease Control and Prevention recently reported that 36% of Americans regularly get less than 7 hours of sleep in a 24-hour period, and that 38% unintentionally fall asleep during the day at least once a month.[7] It thus appears that a significant proportion of us are sleep-deprived, and are probably using caffeine and other stimulants to mask the effects of drowsiness. Given the widespread prevalence of poor sleep health, your struggle with depressed mood might be related to sleep deprivation.

> **Frequent mild sleep loss can contribute to depressed mood.**

Ask yourself these two critical questions:

"Do I often feel tired throughout the day, maybe even unintentionally falling asleep?"

"Do I often experience difficulty concentrating or remembering things because of sleep loss?"

If you answered yes to either question, then sleep disturbance may be contributing significantly to your struggle with depressive mood state. Improving sleep health will be an important mood repair strategy for you.

▶▶▶▶ Repair Strategy 63: Take the Sleep Hygiene Checkup

Our ability to sleep is strongly influenced by our surroundings, because our brains can be conditioned to automatically enter into slumber in the presence of certain cues.

Sleep hygiene refers to the behaviors, practices, and environment that either promote or detract from continuous, effective, and restful sleep.[8] Your goal should be 8 hours of sleep each night. Use the following checklist to determine where you might need to make changes to encourage more restful sleep.

❑ *Are you "multitasking" in bed?* Are you watching TV, using social media, studying, reading, or snacking while lying in bed? You should restrict bed use to sleep or sex, so that the bed becomes a conditioned stimulus for these activities.

❑ *Is your bedtime routine chaotic?* A bedtime routine is preferable to variable waking and sleeping hours. It is best to have a regular bedtime, especially during the week. Set your alarm to wake you up at the same time every morning.

❑ *Are you frequently napping during the day?* There is some controversy about the merits of daytime napping, but it is safe to say that long naps (more than 30 minutes) can reduce the brain's readiness for night sleep if you have sleep difficulties. It's easy to get into a vicious cycle of not sleeping well at night, then napping during the day, followed by a further erosion of sleep readiness at night.

❑ *Is your bedroom too light at night?* A dark bedroom is more conducive to sleep, because sunlight and artificial lighting delay the production of melatonin, which is a sleep-promoting hormone.

❑ *Is your bed or room uncomfortable?* A cool room temperature should be maintained; noises should be reduced, if not eliminated; and the mattress and pillow should be comfortable. Pets may interrupt sleep, as may children or a snoring or "night-roaming" partner.

TOOL FINDER You may need to use the problem-solving strategy presented in Chapter 3 (Repair Strategy 10) to create a more conducive sleep environment for yourself.

❑ *Is exercise interfering in your sleep readiness?* Schedule your exercise so that it contributes to sleep readiness. Exercising 4 or 5 hours before bedtime is optimal for sleep readiness. Evening exercise closer to bedtime might increase arousal and make you less ready for sleep.

❑ *Are you a nighttime "clock watcher"?* If you have difficulty falling asleep, keeping a watch on the clock will increase anxiety and thus delay sleep onset. Turn your alarm clock around so that you can't see the time.

❑ *What are you consuming in the evenings?* If you are having problems falling asleep, consider whether you are consuming any substances that might cause sleep interference. Avoid consuming caffeine after noon, because of its slow rate of body metabolism. Alcohol can disrupt sleep by causing wakefulness in the latter two-thirds of the sleep period. Stimulants (such as nicotine, amphetamines, and herbs like ginseng and ephedra) and certain medications (such as antidepressants, blood pressure medication, anticonvulsants, decongestants, and asthma medications) can also interfere in sleep. If you are taking medications, consult your doctor about their effects on sleep, and make sure you take your medications at the prescribed times.

❑ *Are you lying in bed for hours trying to get to sleep?* You can't force yourself to fall asleep. People often report that they have racing thoughts and worries while trying to sleep; they feel an increase in anxiety and frustration with the elusiveness of sleep. Make sure you go to bed only when you are sleepy. If you can't get to sleep within 30–45 minutes, or you wake up during the night and can't get back to sleep, go to another room and do something boring and relaxing in the dark until you feel sleepy, and then return to bed. Avoid television, the Internet, or reading; all of these introduce light, which stimulates your brain and interferes in melatonin production. There is some disagreement among sleep experts on whether limiting your time in bed when you are not falling asleep is a good idea. The best advice is to try both approaches (i.e., staying in bed vs. getting up) and see what works better for you.

The Sleep Paradox

You can encourage restful sleep by practicing good sleep hygiene; relaxing yourself before bedtime; and using peaceful, calming imagery—but you can't make yourself sleep. Sleep onset is a natural, automatic brain process that defies effortful control. In fact, there is a *paradox* to sleep: The more you try to fall asleep, the less likely you are to experience actual sleep onset. Worry about life concerns will keep you awake, but worry about not sleeping will definitely cause sleep problems. If making changes in basic sleep hygiene doesn't help, try the following strategies.

Use these sleep strategies if you . . .

- become anxious about not falling asleep at night.
- have racing thoughts and worries while trying to fall asleep.
- have put a lot of effort into trying to fall asleep, but have had little success.

▶▶▶ Repair Strategy ⑥④: Adopt a Mindful Approach to Sleeping

The antidote to "sleep worry" is mindful acceptance (see Chapter 7). It is important that you give yourself permission *not* to sleep. The reality is that most of us can deal quite effectively with one or even two nights of lost sleep. We can use different coping skills to deal with the increased fatigue the next day, such as drinking a little extra coffee. There are several steps you can take to use mindful acceptance to help induce sleep. Mindfulness is to be practiced when you first go to bed.

REPAIR STRATEGY 64 INSTRUCTIONS

1. **Give yourself permission to experience less sleep on occasion.** This does not simply mean telling yourself, "It's OK to get only 4 hours of sleep tonight." It means really coming to believe that you can exist on less sleep, and in this way taking the pressure off yourself to fall asleep. One way to do this is to record your daytime experience of reduced sleep. Sure, you felt tired, but did you survive? Were you able to function reasonably well?

2. **Remind yourself that some temporary sleep deprivation will lead to an increase in sleep drive the following night.** Eventually you will fall asleep, so having 1 or 2 reduced sleep nights will increase your sleep readiness the following nights, provided that you don't nap during the day and you follow good sleep hygiene practices.

3. **Remember that you are probably sleeping more than you think.** This means it is not a catastrophe if you don't get the 8 hours of sleep you prefer. Your functioning the next day may not be optimal, but you won't end up in some zombie state either.

4. **As you lie in bed, allow your thoughts to drift through your mind without force, effort, or judgment.** Recall from Chapter 7 that the objective of mindfulness is nonjudgmental acceptance of your thoughts. To achieve this, you must relinquish efforts to control what you are thinking. Often we become frustrated and anxious about not falling asleep, trying to suppress anxious thoughts, and forcing ourselves to think in a calming manner. But this effort at control has the untoward effect of increasing anxiety and preventing sleep onset. *The goal of mindful sleep is to accept in a gentle, nonjudgmental manner your present momentary state of arousal, whether that is full alertness or sleepiness.*

▶ Repair Strategy 65: Redirect Your Attention

You can also attentively focus on "quieting your mind" to deal with sleep worry. This involves redirecting your attention to another engaging, but calming, mental activity.

For example, you could visualize a relaxing scene, recall a pleasant memory, replay scenes from a favorite movie, or play a round of golf or some other favorite sport. Or try thinking about one of your interests, leisure activities, or hobbies (such as gardening, cooking, or woodworking). One of my hobbies is carpentry, and so I do a lot of my own home renovation work. When I am having trouble sleeping, I have found thinking about the various steps in doing a current home renovation project a calming experience. However, this works only because the renovation project is truly a hobby, and so for me it really doesn't have the urgency and importance that thinking about a work deadline would generate. If I were a professional carpenter, thinking about the project might not be so relaxing.

▶ Repair Strategy 66: Try Controlled Breathing or Progressive Relaxation

There are various relaxation strategies that can be used to achieve a quiet, calm state conducive to sleep. One of these is called *controlled diaphragmatic breathing*. This is similar to the focus on the breath in mindfulness meditation as described in Chapter 7. Instructions on diaphragmatic breathing can be found on a webpage maintained by the American Medical Student Association (*www.amsa.org/healingthehealer/breathing.cfm*) and another maintained by the University of Texas Counseling and Mental Health Center (*www.cmhc.utexas.edu/stressrecess/Level_Two/breathing.html*).

Or you could try *progressive muscle relaxation*, which involves tensing and relaxing various muscle groups. Webpages maintained by AnxietyBC (*www.anxietybc.com/sites/default/files/CalmBreathing.pdf*) and MindTools (*www.mindtools.com/stress/RelaxationTechniques/PhysicalTechniques.htm*) offer step-by-step instructions for doing progressive muscle relaxation.

Diet and Mood

No doubt you have heard the phrase "You are what you eat," and this appears to apply to your mood state as well. Although there is great controversy, as well as many exaggerated claims, about the influence of certain types of food on physical and mental health, there is some evidence that a so-called "Mediterranean" dietary pattern, and possibly a dietary supplement of omega-3 fatty acids, can be helpful in lowering risk for depression. In a 4-year study involving over 10,000 Spanish university students, adherence to a Mediterranean dietary pattern was associated with a lower risk of clinical depression.[9] This dietary pattern includes (1) a high intake of monounsaturated fatty acids (e.g., olive oil), legumes (e.g., beans, peas), fruit and nuts, fish, cereals (e.g., bread), and vegetables; (2) a moderate intake of milk and dairy products, as well as red wine; and (3) a low intake of meat and meat products.

Diet can also have indirect effects on negative mood through weight gain and obesity. For many individuals, being overweight or obese is a significant contributor to increased problems with depressed mood. To the extent that poor diet may be a major factor in unwanted weight gain, this represents another pathway in which food intake affects feelings.

⟫⟫⟫➡ Repair Strategy 67: Make Dietary Changes

Take a look at your daily diet, and consider how well it matches the Mediterranean dietary pattern. If you are eating a lot of processed foods, red meat, salty foods, and/or sugar-saturated foods, and then experiencing additional unwanted weight gain, your dietary habits may be having a greater impact on your emotional health than you think.

You may want to consider consulting with a dietitian to formulate a dietary plan that promotes healthy living. This could have a major impact on your mood state, help you maintain a healthy weight range, and supply you with the fuel (i.e., energy) you need to pursue your exercise program.

If you are interested in weight loss, I would recommend the Beck Diet Solution, created by Judith S. Beck and Deborah Beck Busis (for more information, see *www.beckdietsolution.com*).

TOOL FINDER Being motivated to make major lifestyle changes is one of the biggest challenges we all face. If you are having difficulty with motivation for physical activity even after working on the previous mood repair exercise strategies, consult the following chapters:

- Chapter 7 on making behavioral changes
- Chapter 9 on goal setting
- Chapter 13 on avoidance and procrastination

13 face your dread

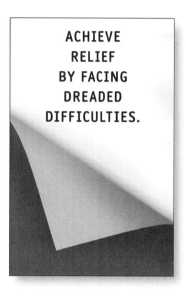

ACHIEVE RELIEF BY FACING DREADED DIFFICULTIES.

Juanita had graduated from college with top honors and was now employed as a supervisor with a multinational insurance company. Although she was a fairly recent hire, Juanita had risen quickly through the ranks. She was an outstanding customer relations officer and soon won a number of awards for her excellent service. She was offered two promotions that took her into middle management. Juanita prided herself on having a strong work ethic, ambition, and intelligence. She had a promising future with the company, and her life generally seemed to be going well.

Although Juanita was a high achiever, she had always struggled with depressed feelings, especially after a disappointment or failure. Throughout college her moods had fluctuated dramatically, depending on her exam grades. She'd tried to lift herself out of despair, but often the only way her mood would improve was if she happened to do better on another exam. When she got into a funk after doing poorly on a test, she would often spend several days avoiding classes or study. She then got further behind in her work, which made it difficult to prepare for her next exams. Juanita had serious problems in dealing with failure, and her tendency to avoid situations of anticipated failure only made the situation worse.

At work, her first major disappointment was failure to receive the "junior manager of the year" award—a recognition she'd received every year since her promotion to a managerial position. This came as quite a blow, and Juanita was soon filled with the self-doubts, criticism, and negativity that had haunted her as a student. Her mood plummeted, and she started missing her performance targets. Asked to appear before the managerial review committee, she was told that the decline in her performance had been noticed, and concern was expressed about her future with the company. Juanita left that meeting fearful and discouraged. She realized she was now being watched and could lose her job if she didn't improve. But rather than reinvigorating her work performance, the meeting had the opposite effect: Juanita felt more and more apprehensive, sank deeper into doubt about her ability to do the job, and became more anxious and depressed. She started dreading the end of the weekend and the return of the work week.

After several weeks, Juanita went to her family doctor, who recommended that she take stress leave from work, begin a trial of antidepressants, and see a mental health therapist for psychotherapy. Juanita agreed to all these recommendations, but now, after 3 months on short-term disability, she was dreading the return to work. As the end of her disability leave approached, Juanita noticed that she was becoming more and more agitated and depressed. How could she possibly cope with the demands of work? What would people think of her for taking a stress leave? What if her employer was impatient and fired her soon after she returned to work? How could she face her family and friends? Juanita was plagued with worries about her return to work. This was one problem she would love to avoid at all costs.

Difficulties, adversities, and disappointments are all too often part of the human existence. Unfortunately, people who struggle with low moods have a higher rate of negative life stressors, especially events involving humiliation, entrapment, loss, danger, social defeat, rejection, and exclusion. Add the negativity that plagues those prone to depression, and opting for avoidance or even denial, rather than dealing directly with adversities and life problems, is understandable. Sadly, however, avoidance often just makes these problems worse—and a vicious cycle develops, in which the negative effects of the life problem intensify over time, leading to ever-deeper depression and despair. Procrastination and other forms of avoidance, therefore, are powerful negative forces. They can be both causes and consequences of low mood: When people avoid what they fear, they feel more depressed; but when they feel depressed, they turn more easily to avoidance.

Avoidance may have become a dominant coping strategy in your life; that is, you may frequently put off or avoid a variety of problems or situations. Or there may be one or two big issues in your life that you avoid. Juanita struggled with both types of avoidance. She tended to put off or otherwise avoid any difficult task that she sensed might lead to failure, and she had difficulty facing a transition connected with a major source of perceived failure in her life—her return to work after stress leave. The strategies presented in this chapter will help you overcome both types of avoidance: the generalized type and the more specific avoidance of a major life problem.

Use the strategies for dealing with procrastination and other forms of avoidance if you . . .

- generally engage in avoidance to cope with difficult and unpleasant experiences.
- consider yourself a procrastinator.

- dread facing one or two major life issues or problems.
- trace your struggle with low mood to unresolved problems or issues.

Why Do We Avoid Things?

Avoidance is choosing a course of action (or inaction) that brings immediate relief, rather than a more adaptive behavior that may cause immediate distress but is more helpful in the long term.[1] For example, Ranjit, a college student, may choose watching TV over studying because he feels anxious and discouraged about his performance in a course. So watching TV brings immediate relief and he avoids the distress of studying, even though in the long run he'll do better on the exam if he studies and worse on the exam if he keeps watching TV. The mantra for the avoidant person is "short-term gain [distress relief], but long-term pain [persistence and escalation of distress]." *Procrastination* is a type of avoidance; it involves voluntarily delaying the initiation or completion of an intended course of action, even though you expect to be worse off in the future for the delay.[2] Although procrastination is extremely common, and we know it's a bad idea, it can be a really hard habit to break. In all

> **Procrastination and other types of avoidance fuel depression via a short-sighted focus on immediate relief.**

my years of clinical work, I've never met a person who mistakenly thought procrastination was helpful. So why do we persist in our procrastination and other avoidance, especially when we are feeling down?

▸▸▸▸ Repair Strategy 68:
Complete a Procrastination/Avoidance Checklist

The first step in getting a handle on your procrastination and other forms of avoidance is to know why you engage in these behaviors. The reasons in the following checklist may seem obvious in some cases, but that doesn't make them any less potent in fueling the behaviors, so it's good to bring them to the surface where you can deal with them. As you go through this checklist, think about a problem or issue in your life that through continued avoidance makes you feel more depressed (e.g., organizing your personal finances, dealing with a difficult or unreasonable child, ongoing marital strain and conflict, poor health, unreasonable work demands).

❑ *Do you avoid difficult or unpleasant tasks?* Although we are all more likely to put off or otherwise avoid unpleasant or difficult tasks, not everyone reacts to difficulty in the same way. Some people actually seem to thrive on difficulty, viewing it as a challenge. But if you're overly concerned about failure, you might tend to misjudge the difficulty and unpleasantness of tasks and so avoid them. To take a personal finance example, you're more likely to view income tax or bill paying as difficult if money is tight. So you procrastinate, but of course the bills don't disappear; they only get worse if not dealt with properly. The worse your financial situation is, the more distressed you become. *Do you postpone or avoid many responsibilities in your life because you misjudge them as overly difficult and unpleasant?*

❑ *Do you expect failure?* If you don't expect to succeed at a task, or you believe that you don't have the skills or ability necessary to achieve a successful outcome, you're more likely to procrastinate or avoid it. Again, people differ in their tendency to predict failure. It may have become so natural for you to have thoughts and beliefs about your inability to succeed that you're hardly aware of them.

❑ *Is it hard for you to visualize success in dealing with an issue?* Let's say you've been concerned about your adult son's unemployment and attitude toward work. If you can't see yourself being able to talk to him about his unemployment, you're likely to give up and avoid having the talk. The problem only gets worse, and you feel more helpless and down about the situation.

❑ *Do you tend to put things off, and then to do them at the last possible minute?* We are all more likely to procrastinate when a deadline is farther in the future. It is easier to put off working on taxes in mid-February than it is in mid-April. This problem may be compounded by the cognitive error of *short-sightedness* (see Chapter 12), which involves misjudging the amount of time available to complete a job in the future. As a university professor, I see this with every course I teach. I assign a 10-page essay at the beginning of each term, but few students get the paper in early, even though they could obtain bonus points for early submission. Instead, they wait until the end of the term, when they are much busier with exams and other assignments.

❑ *Do you have problems with organization that cause you to neglect some of your daily responsibilities?* Procrastination and other avoidance behaviors come more naturally to certain types of people—people who are more distractible, struggle more with organization, and have greater difficulty being goal-directed.[2] If this describes you, then working on your procrastination/avoidance problems may be especially challenging. Even though you'll be trying to change lifelong habits, you can expect to make improvements if you use the strategies presented in this chapter.

❑ *Do you often feel too fatigued to make the necessary effort?* How often have you said to yourself, "I'm too tired to try, so why bother?" I meet often with procrastinating students and can often hear the fatigue in their voices. We are all more likely to procrastinate during depressed moods, and this is caused primarily by the lethargy or lack of energy that accompanies feeling blue. If low energy contributes to your procrastination, you should consult with your family doctor to ensure that no underlying medical condition or clinical depression accounts for your malaise.

❑ *Do you tend to think of the worst-case scenario when you are confronted with a difficult or unpleasant task?* Catastrophizing, or imagining the worst possible outcome to a situation, will increase apprehension and so encourage you to delay action. If you predict that you'll have a big tax bill and won't be able to pay it, you will be more likely to postpone filing your income tax. Thinking the worst is self-defeating, because it only increases anxiety and worry, and only rarely does the worst ever happen. More often, a moderately negative outcome occurs—one that you can deal with quite effectively. Confronting your imagined catastrophe may be important to getting yourself started on an avoided task or issue.

❑ *Do you have difficulty expressing negative emotions, preferring to suppress (i.e., avoid) anger, frustration, fear, or sadness?* The situations, tasks, and other life problems people avoid are often associated with a variety of negative emotions that can be highly unpleasant. For example, imagine that you said something against a coworker that you later found out was not true. You realize that you need to speak to the coworker you offended, offer an apology, and attempt to mend the broken relationship. It may also necessitate a meeting with your supervisor to clear the air at the office. However, you find yourself putting off doing the right thing. Maybe you're anticipating a confrontation, or maybe you don't want to experience the increased feelings of shame, guilt, embarrassment, and humiliation that could come with speaking directly with the offended coworker. And so you suffer through the immediate feelings of guilt and despair associated with your avoidance of the offended person, because you expect attempts at reconciliation to make you feel even worse.

❑ *Do you lack confidence in your decision making, often worrying that you'll make a mistake?* Indecision is another feature of depression, and often procrastination or other avoidance is caused by not knowing which course of action should be taken in a given situation. The indecision can be driven by a need to be certain of the outcome, a fear of making a mistake, being overly focused on short-term goals, or demanding an unrealistic level of reassurance. If you are dithering, then delay can make you feel as if a decision has been averted. But of course procrastination and other forms of avoidance *are* decisions; they involve choosing short-term goals over a long-term healthier solution. So deciding to watch TV rather than work on your income tax is a decision, even if you tell yourself, "I'm not working on my income tax because I can't decide what to claim as an expense."

❑ *Do you feel a sense of relief when you delay a dreaded task?* Have you ever had to make a telephone call that you were dreading? Finally, after considerable delay, you muster the courage and make the call, only to find that the person does not answer. Have you noticed the immediate sense of relief you felt when no one answered, even though it is short-lived? Feeling relief from heightened anxiety is a positive emotional experience. Avoiding work on a difficult and aversive task can bring a temporary sense of relief that reinforces procrastination, but there's nothing like the genuine relief that comes with resolving a difficult situation.

❑ *Are you easily bored?* Sometimes people postpone or avoid tasks they perceive as boring by distracting themselves with more pleasant short-term activities. In fact, people differ greatly in their tolerance for boredom and need for novelty or excitement. Working on income taxes, studying, writing up the minutes of a business meeting, doing housework, and organizing the garage are all activities that few people find interesting. So a low tolerance for uninteresting tasks may cause you to choose more exciting short-term options, such as going to the movies, playing sports, visiting with friends, or shopping. The problem is that these short-term distractions cause a delay in completing highly important but uninteresting work.

Having identified the reasons for your procrastination and other forms of avoidance, you are now ready to take a strategic approach to breaking these patterns. Unlike in other chapters, the strategies presented below are interrelated. You will want to use these strategies together as a package to deal with the more specific problems of avoidance and delay. Knowing the reasons why you procrastinate and otherwise avoid things, identifying their sources, setting goals, and implementing a behavioral plan of action are all strategies you'll need to use to break the grip of these problems.

⟫⟫⟫➡ Repair Strategy ⓺⓽: Identify Your Procrastination/Avoidance Patterns

To *dread* something means to feel fear or apprehension about facing something, so people frequently try to avoid dreaded situations, tasks, and circumstances. The first step in changing procrastination and other types of avoidance, therefore, is to know what you dread and how you are avoiding it (or them). Have these behaviors been lifelong problems causing interference in a variety of daily functions, or have you been avoiding one or two major issues? Whether you are a "generalized" or "specific" avoider, the effects of avoidance on negative mood will be the same. You can identify what you're avoiding by using the Procrastination/Avoidance Record shown in part on the next page, or print out a complete one from *www.guilford.com/clark7-forms*.

Procrastination/Avoidance Record

Personal problem, situation, or task procrastinated/avoided	Reasons for procrastination/ avoidance	Consequences of procrastination/ avoidance
1.		
2.		

REPAIR STRATEGY 69 INSTRUCTIONS

1. **Take time to reflect upon the last few weeks, and enter any tasks, problems, situations, or responsibilities associated with procrastination or other types of avoidance in the Procrastination/Avoidance Record.** The things you are avoiding in your life could be minor daily tasks or responsibilities, or they could be major life issues or problems. Maybe you've tended to put off these things all your life, or maybe they are more recent difficulties because of the blues you've been stuck in lately. Ask a friend or family member to help you complete the record if you're having trouble identifying your procrastination/avoidance behavior.

2. **Review the record and look for recurrent patterns of procrastination/avoidance. Do one or two specific issues appear to dominate these behaviors, or is a general theme emerging?**

3. **Examine the consequences.** As you read over the final column in the form, what are the detrimental effects of avoidance and delay? Are there negative consequences for your work, finances, relationships, or health—consequences that will make your life situation even worse? Are these behaviors having direct effects on your mood state, making you feel more depressed, guilty, or embarrassed?

4. **Prioritize your work on procrastination/avoidance.** Rearrange the situations or tasks recorded in the first column into a list, starting with the most important and working down to the least important. The postponed/avoided situation or task that has the greatest negative impact on your emotional well-being should be at the top of the list. You will want to begin your plan for breaking the grip of procrasti-

nation and other types of avoidance in your daily living by targeting the situations that have the greatest impact on your mood state.

To illustrate, let's look at the Procrastination/Avoidance Record (see next page) filled out by Juanita, who was dreading returning to work after taking a short-term disability leave for work stress, and who struggled with procrastination and avoidance in other areas of her life that contributed to her being stuck in the blues.

Juanita forgot that she had been putting off working on her personal finances, and doing nothing all day but sit around the house watching reality TV shows, playing computer games, or checking social media, until she talked to her parents one evening about her recent struggles with procrastination. Reviewing her Procrastination/Avoidance Record, Juanita realized that perceived or anticipated failure played a huge role in her behavior. She noticed that anticipated unpleasantness, expectation of failure, catastrophizing, and short-sightedness were major contributors to her avoidance: Whenever she thought she might fail at something, she would avoid or delay dealing with it. This was a lifelong pattern, but it got much worse when she was feeling depressed. It was evident that she needed to work on dealing with situations involving a perceived risk of failure. Because the consequences of avoiding work and bill paying were much greater than the argument with her friend, Juanita decided to focus on breaking these avoidance issues and to leave the argument with her friend to a later time.

⟫⟫⟫➡ Repair Strategy ⓻⓪: Set Short-Term Goals for Overcoming Procrastination/Avoidance

Once you've selected a problem from your Procrastination/Avoidance Record, you can break the problem down into a series of more manageable steps, setting specific short-term goals at each step.

REPAIR STRATEGY 70 INSTRUCTIONS

1. **Set clearly defined goals.**

> **TOOL FINDER** Review Chapters 5 and 9 (Repair Strategies 19 and 36, respectively) for more extensive discussions of goal setting.

2. **Make sure the goals are achievable within a day or so; they should extend no more than a week ahead.** If the goals are too lofty or set too far into the future, you will be more likely to procrastinate.

Procrastination/Avoidance Record: Juanita

Personal problem, situation, or task procrastinated/avoided	Reasons for procrastination/avoidance	Consequences of procrastination/avoidance
1. I need to set up a meeting with my supervisor, disability rep, and therapist to get my return-to-work process started, but I haven't sent the email to schedule this meeting.	I view the task as unpleasant. I expect to fail to keep my job; I keep thinking the outcome will be the worst.	The anxiety and apprehension about returning to work are getting worse. I'm becoming more convinced I'll lose my job no matter what I do. Delaying contact is only making me feel more depressed and believe that my life is ruined.
2. I haven't looked at my bills or checking account for weeks.	Again, the task is unpleasant. I engage in short-sightedness. I feel relief at not dealing with the bills.	I'm going further into debt. I'm paying high interest charges on credit cards. I end up listening to belligerent calls from credit card companies. My life feels out of control.
3. I had a serious argument with my best friend about work, and now I'm avoiding any contact with her.	Short-sightedness; difficulty expressing negative emotion.	I feel intense loneliness. I've had more tearful episodes about having no friends. I feel guilty for what I said to Betty and realize I'll lose a good friend if I don't apologize. I'm losing confidence in my socializing ability, and now I question whether people even like me.

Juanita realized that she could no longer delay starting her return-to-work process if she wanted to keep her job. Because she lacked sufficient energy and motivation to get started, she decided that the first task was to talk to her therapist about formulating an action plan for getting this process underway. This was set for her next appointment in 3 days. At the therapy session, Juanita and her therapist decided that the next step was to send an email to her work disability consultant saying that she intended to email her supervisor for a return-to-work meeting. She would complete this task in 2 days. Depending on the advice of her disability consultant, she would then email her supervisor for a meeting by the end of the week. The next therapy session would focus on rehearsing communication and anxiety management skills Juanita could use during her meeting with the supervisor. If the meeting with the supervisor led to a firm return-to-work date, Juanita wanted to contact a couple of close coworkers and take them to lunch, informing them of her intention to return. She felt it was important to have some social support in place to help her get through the first few days back at work.

Whenever Juanita thought about returning to work, she immediately avoided the issue, because she had lost confidence in her ability to handle stress (i.e., she had low self-efficacy beliefs); she believed that eventually she would be fired because of her "mental weakness" (i.e., she was catastrophizing); and she anticipated that she would feel shame and embarrassment around her coworkers who knew she had taken stress leave. By breaking the problem down into a series of steps with specific short-term goals, Juanita could focus on these goals rather than on the overwhelming bigger picture. As discussed in Chapter 7, it is critical to focus on the present—"What is the next thing I need to do today?"—rather than letting your mind race ahead into the future. Breaking a formidable problem into smaller steps and setting short-term, realistic goals can have a positive effect on daily mood by reminding you that you're making progress toward dealing with the dreaded problem.

▸▸▸▸ Repair Strategy **71**: Create Alternatives

Behavioral activation therapy emphasizes the importance of shifting from TRAP (Trigger, Response, Avoidance Pattern) to TRAC (Trigger, Response, Alternative Coping).[1] Instead of engaging in a semiautomatic avoidance response whenever you are reminded of a problem or task, you can have at your disposal more adaptive coping responses that help you actually resolve the difficult situation. These alternative coping behaviors should be used to block procrastination/avoidance behavior and encourage you to work on the dreaded task or problem. You can employ these coping responses to achieve the goals you have set in using Repair Strategy 70.

REPAIR STRATEGY 71 INSTRUCTIONS

1. **Review your goal-setting plan, and list all the specific steps you need to take to counter procrastination and avoidance.** In Juanita's action plan for starting her return-to-work process, the various steps involved talking to her therapist about the return-to-work issue, emailing her supervisor for a meeting, rehearsing communication and anxiety management skills with her therapist, and inviting a couple of coworker friends to lunch.

2. **With each step, describe what you need to do—that is, what behaviors you need to implement to succeed at that step.** Again, Juanita realized she needed to be more assertive. First, she actually asked her therapist to spend time in the session dealing with the return-to-work issue. In regard to emailing her supervisor, she decided to write a draft email and seek feedback from her brother on the appropriateness of her message, given his experience in human resource issues.

3. **Give yourself a strict time limit for engaging in each alternative behavior.** Since delay is the key ingredient in procrastination, you will need to be strict, giving yourself a specific time and date when you will complete the behavior. You could use accountability or reward yourself with some enjoyable activity for completing the behavior. Emailing her supervisor was a big hurdle for Juanita, so she told her parents and brother that she would email him by Friday. She also decided to go out to a movie Friday night once she accomplished the task.

> **TOOL FINDER**   Use the ACTION plans presented in Chapter 5 (see Repair Strategy 20) to develop your approach for staying on track and not being derailed by procrastination or other types of avoidance.

4. **Evaluate the outcome of the alternative coping behavior.** After completing the alternative behavior, take time to evaluate the outcome. How successful was the new behavior? Did the problem get resolved? Do you feel you made some progress on the issue you've been avoiding? What impact has this had on your mood state? Was dealing with the problem more or less difficult than you expected? By evaluating the success of your alternative behavior plan, you will increase your confidence in dealing with problems or difficult situations rather than avoiding them.

In another example of using TRAC, Juanita constructed a list of alternative behaviors to block other avoidance responses, such as sleeping, playing computer games, or telling herself she'd "do it tomorrow." Each morning before playing computer games, she would read all the email announcements from work; she would always answer the telephone; and she would give a brief reply of acknowledgment indicating she had received any work emails sent to her personally. She would also take her driving route to work at least twice a week, to increase exposure to work-related cues that might cause anxiety. At least three times a week she would read over past reports she had completed before her stress leave, to familiarize herself with the work she had done in the past. Eventually Juanita started having email contact with a couple of close coworkers and actually met them for lunch once or twice before returning to work. Notice that all of these activities were alternatives to Juanita's typical procrastination/ avoidance behaviors. So the key idea is to stay on TRAC in dealing with dread, rather than to fall into the TRAP of delay and avoidance.

▸▸▸▸ Repair Strategy **72**: Replace "Can't Do" with "Can Do"

Chapter 4 has discussed how negative thinking increases depressed mood and how you can counter this thinking to improve your mood state. Negative thoughts and beliefs are also found in procrastination and other forms of avoidance. The main belief in these instances is helplessness: "I'm too weak. I just can't face this problem. There's no sense in trying; I will only feel worse. I'll try to do something later." The problem is that such negative, defeatist thinking will strengthen avoidance patterns and under-mine coping efforts. It will also reinforce expectations of failure, catastrophizing, and lack of confidence in decision making—all factors that you may have checked off on the checklist in Repair Strategy 68.

Use Repair Strategy 72 particularly if . . .

- you're feeling very discouraged about the dreaded or avoided problem.
- you're blaming yourself or feeling you are responsible for the situation you now avoid.
- you consider yourself weak or lazy for not dealing with the dreaded issue.

REPAIR STRATEGY 72 INSTRUCTIONS

1. **Become aware of your negative thinking.** When procrastination and other types of avoidance are causing substantial problems in your life, it is easy to become focused on the maladaptive behavior and not recognize the dysfunctional think-ing that may be driving the avoidance. Knowing your "procrastination mindset" is an important step in your battle to overcome delay and avoidance.

2. **Use the cognitive strategies discussed in Chapter 4 to arrive at a more realis-tic, adaptive perspective on the avoided task or dreaded situation.** Once you've identified the thoughts and beliefs underlying your procrastination/avoidance, you can tailor the cognitive strategies in Chapter 4 to counter this specific type

of negative thinking. No doubt the main belief you will need to correct with the cognitive strategies is the expectation that something terrible is going to happen and you are helpless to deal with it.

TOOL FINDER Evaluating the evidence for and against avoidance-related thinking (Repair Strategy 12); becoming more aware of the biases in how you view the problem (Repair Strategy 13); generating an alternative perspective on the difficult situation (Repair Strategy 14); and then taking action that challenges negative thinking (Repair Strategy 16) are all useful cognitive strategies for developing a coping-oriented attitude to your problems.

3. **In your search for evidence that you are not as helpless as you think, try to recall how you (and others) have coped with similar difficulties in the past.** What was the long-term outcome, and how well have you adjusted to these past circumstances? Do you have any close friends or family members who have gone through similar difficulties? Is there anything you can learn from them about the best coping strategies? When feeling depressed, you may often forget about your own and others' past successes. Reminding yourself of successful coping with past difficulties can bolster your confidence to face the problems of today that you are avoiding.

Whenever Juanita thought about contacting someone from work, she immediately became overwhelmed with fear and apprehension. Negative, avoidant thoughts flooded her mind, such as "I'm feeling so upset; clearly I'm not ready to go back to work," "I've lost all my confidence; I'm not the strong person I was in the past," and "I'm still emotionally fragile; if I try to deal with work, I'm going to have a relapse." This type of thinking served as a powerful reinforcement for procrastination. However, in doing the cognitive work discussed in Chapter 4, Juanita was reminded of a similar incident in her junior year of college. She was taking several difficult courses, and despite intense study, she was not getting the grades she expected. She started to slip into depression and was advised to withdraw from the semester by a counselor at Student Services. She recalled that after working with the counselor on several coping strategies, she returned to college the next semester and obtained the highest semester GPA in her entire undergraduate program. Recalling this university experience helped Juanita challenge her negative, avoidant thinking about work; it provided concrete evidence that she could successfully cope with a dreaded situation.

⫸ Repair Strategy 🅱: Manipulate Environmental Cues

Another way to reduce procrastination/avoidance and encourage adaptive coping is through a process called *stimulus control*. Essentially, this involves restructuring your environment so that it confronts you with cues that confirm your goals, rather than with reminders of distracting, avoidant behaviors.[2] In other words, you can structure your environment so that it takes less effort to engage in coping behavior and more effort to engage in avoidance behavior. This can be a powerful strategy for encouraging adaptive coping, because energy is already in short supply when you are feeling depressed.

Use Repair Strategy 73 particularly if . . .

- your procrastination is caused by boredom.
- you experience relief as a result of delay.
- your avoidance is due to short-sightedness.

REPAIR STRATEGY 73 INSTRUCTIONS

1. **Review the Procrastination/Avoidance Record (see Repair Strategy 69), paying particular attention to the first two columns of this form.** Write down a description of your procrastination and other avoidance behavior associated with each situation. How do you procrastinate? Is your living environment structured in a manner that facilitates or even encourages avoidant and distracting behavior? Juanita, for example, realized that she tended to "goof off" on her computer and watch TV rather than deal with any work-related issues. Her laptop and TV were both in her bedroom, so it was easy to get involved in both distractions without even getting out of bed. She realized she was spending hours in her room surfing the Internet, playing games, or watching TV. All of these activities were much too easily accessible to her.

2. **Think about what would facilitate your alternative coping behavior.** Take a critical look at your living space, and see whether you could rearrange it to make the coping behavior easier and the avoidant behavior more difficult. For example, maybe you know you should be calling friends and family members in order to improve your social connections (see Chapter 10). But instead you get caught up in listening to music or checking Facebook. You could rearrange your apartment so that the landline phone is more accessible, and your smartphone, with all its

distracting features, is turned off and stored away in a drawer. This would encourage you to use the landline and make the phone calls you intend to make.

3. **Make the environmental changes that will reduce avoidant behavior and increase coping behavior.** Juanita noted that she would lie in bed most of the morning checking social media and playing computer games on her laptop. She decided to get up earlier in the morning to an alarm, make the bed, shower, and eat breakfast before checking her computer. Also, she would power down the computer in the evening, so that it was offline when she woke up in the morning. After breakfast she could boot up the computer, but she could view it only in the room she used as an office. She would confine her viewing time to 1 hour and would read two or three work-related emails before engaging in more pleasurable computer activities.

Repair Strategy 74: Create Contingent Rewards

One of the best ways to encourage healthy coping responses is to pair them with something pleasurable or rewarding. Working on your action plan for dealing with a dreaded situation or avoided task will be difficult, so you will need to reward yourself when you do engage in coping behavior.

Use Repair Strategy 74 especially if . . .

- you've made several false starts in breaking the grip of procrastination/avoidance.
- you're having difficulty with motivation.
- you've lost interest in dealing with the dreaded problem or situation.

REPAIR STRATEGY 74 INSTRUCTIONS

1. **Make a commitment to work on your short-term goals.** Review your Procrastination/Avoidance Record (Repair Strategy 69) to select a specific situation or problem for attention. Then consult the goals you set for yourself in Repair Strategy 70, together with the action plan you created in Repair Strategy 71.
2. **Organize the various steps in your action plan in a graded fashion, so you begin with coping behaviors that are least difficult and work up to coping activities that are much more difficult.** For example, Juanita started her action plan by discussing a return to work with her therapist; then she contacted her disability consultant; and then she emailed her supervisor about a meeting. and began checking

mass emails related to work. Notice that Juanita not only broke down the problem of work-related avoidance into more manageable chunks, but also arranged the work in a *graded hierarchy*. That is, she started with an easier, less distressing task and worked her way up to more threatening activities.

3. **At each step along this hierarchy of coping, reward yourself when you stick to the schedule and complete a task.** The reward does not have to be large or expensive; even small pleasures can encourage adaptive behavior. You can pair a short-term pleasant activity with a longer-term adaptive behavior.

   Let's say you've been avoiding work on your income tax. You've broken it down into a series of steps, but you know that the first step is to find last year's returns and locate your income statements from your employer. You also need to set up a place at home where you'll work on your tax return. So you schedule a time to engage in these activities, which you decide will be Monday night right after supper. You'll spend 1 hour on the task and then, as a reward, watch some basketball on TV—a highly pleasurable event. If you don't do the income tax work, you must not watch the game. This is the only way that rewarding contingencies can be used effectively to break avoidance and procrastination. You will need to be disciplined with yourself, engaging in the pleasurable activity only when you've completed a task related to your action plan.

   You might find it helpful to have a list of pleasurable activities that you can consult when you want to reward yourself for coping behavior. It's important to use a variety of rewards, and to make sure you reserve some of these pleasant activities for times when you've completed your coping work.

TOOL FINDER You've already done this work in Chapter 5 (Repair Strategies 17 and 18), so you could consult your Hourly Behavior Record to select highly enjoyable activities to use as contingent rewards. (As noted in Chapter 5, you can also consult various predetermined lists of pleasant events that can be found online.)

4. **In addition to giving yourself tangible rewards for coping behavior, it is important that you exercise loving kindness and compassion toward yourself as you struggle to cope with a dreaded and avoided situation.**

TOOL FINDER See Chapter 11 for details on self-compassion.

Breaking through any form of avoidance is hard work; it takes great effort, even courage, to face what you have been avoiding. So when you do accomplish a step in your action plan, congratulate yourself. It may be a small step, but you are heading in the right direction. You need to revel in the fact that you are doing something about the problem. Berating yourself, discounting your accomplishment, or dismissing your efforts as inconsequential will not promote adaptive coping. It will only breed negativity, discouragement, and despair—factors that will plunge you back into procrastination and other types of avoidance.

Breaking the Grip of Procrastination/Avoidance

Although most people report that they occasionally procrastinate, up to 20% of the general population are chronic procrastinators.[2] Whether procrastination and other forms of avoidance are serious problems or minor inconveniences, people readily acknowledge their harmful effects and wish to reduce these behaviors. For individuals struggling with the blues, the problems of procrastination and avoidance are greatly intensified. Fatigue, loss of interest, passivity, and negative thinking (about the self, the world, and the future) can all amplify the tendency to delay and avoid. This tendency may even extend to engaging in healthy lifestyle behaviors, such as physical exercise, sleep, balanced diet, and socializing; even though these are excellent mood repair strategies, you may be struggling to do them. In this way, an avoidant behavioral pattern can contribute both directly and indirectly to increased sadness. Breaking the grip of procrastination and other types of avoidance will be an important mood repair approach for many people with depressive mood. The strategies presented in this chapter should help you to pursue this approach; no doubt, however, you will have to draw on mood repair strategies presented in other chapters as well.

TOOL FINDER

- Chapter 2 can help you time your work on behavioral changes to coincide with the natural fluctuations in your mood state.
- Consult Chapter 5 on behavioral change as you work specifically on delay and avoidant behavior.
- If your avoidance often involves social situations, review Chapter 10.
- Above all, consult Chapter 11 to remind yourself how to practice self-compassion as you attempt to change entrenched and self-defeating behavioral patterns.

14 sing in the rain

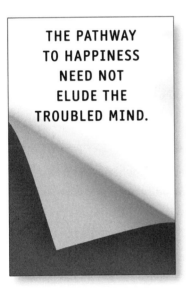

THE PATHWAY TO HAPPINESS NEED NOT ELUDE THE TROUBLED MIND.

If happiness, joy, and contentment depended on living a trouble-free life, then inner peace and life satisfaction would elude us all. Fortunately, this is not the case. Although annual polls show that most people experience minor stressful events each year, and that large numbers of people experience less frequent major stressors (e.g., deaths, divorces, and job losses), over 90% of Americans rate themselves as generally "very happy" or "quite happy."[1] Happiness, it appears, can coexist quite comfortably with life's losses, dangers, disappointments, and failures. You may have days when sadness and despair overtake you, but you can still experience great joy and accomplishment on other days. As noted in Chapter 2, there is a daily ebb and flow to emotions.

When people are asked whether they generally feel positive or negative emotion, or whether they are feeling positive or negative emotion at this moment, the two types are not strongly related to each other except when people are in a stressful condition. What this means is that happiness and sadness need to be treated as different emotional states. Eliminating sadness will not automatically make you happy. For sure, you will feel less sad, but you still may not feel happy. To experience happiness or other positive mood states, you will need to use emotion strategies that directly build these states.

Sadness and happiness are distinct emotion states, each requiring its own emotion regulation strategies.

Most of us in North America live as if we believe wealth and material possessions are the routes to happiness and well-being. Our capitalist economic system puts an incredible emphasis on wealth generation and material success. Over several decades, the effect of economic prosperity on the happiness of entire populations has been researched intensely by social scientists. It turns out that the relationship between income, material possessions, and standard of living on the one hand, and happiness and fulfillment on the other, is complex. The acquisition of more wealth, at least in the developed world, does not necessarily lead to more happiness. After a satiation point is reached where most material needs are met, which is the situation of most middle-class North Americans, it takes an ever-greater amount of earnings to achieve an ever-diminishing increase in life satisfaction. One reason for this is what is called the *hedonic treadmill*. This term refers to the finding that when people experience an increase in income, they quickly adapt to the new income and revert to a preexisting level of happiness.[1] For example, I might feel great for a while after receiving a 20% salary increase, but soon my spending will also increase, and I'll revert to the same emotions I had before I got the increase. And yet so many of us work so hard for better jobs, promotions, and better salaries, thinking, "If I could just earn more, I would be so much happier." It turns out that nothing could be further from the truth. So the old adage "Money doesn't bring happiness" has been supported scientifically. Devoting so much of our lives to generating more and more wealth is a poor investment for happiness and life satisfaction. What, then, is the pathway to happiness?

> There is scientific evidence that more wealth and higher status do not produce greater increases in happiness.

In the last several years, research on the nature of happiness (as defined in the next section) has begun to provide some answers to this question. We now know of an approach to life that increases the frequency and duration of positive emotion. I call these *mood enhancement* strategies, because they seek to prolong positive emotion. All of this book so far has focused on *mood repair* in order to reduce negative mood, or sadness. If you are stuck in the blues, you'll want to first spend time on strategies that decrease depressed mood. But you probably want to experience not just less negative mood, but also more positive mood—more happiness, joy, and fulfillment. So you need to consider mood enhancement strategies as well.

The Pursuit of Happiness

Throughout the ages, prophets, mystics, philosophers, theologians, physicians, and now social scientists have offered up a variety of terms and definitions to capture the essence of the "good life." Our present focus, however, is on one specific aspect of life satisfaction—the experience of positive mood or happiness. So, for the purposes of this chapter, *happiness* is defined as a momentary emotion state in which you feel pleasurably engaged in a situation or activity through which your personal efforts lead to progress toward attaining a desired goal.

This definition may sound like a mouthful, but think back to the last time you felt truly happy. What was that experience like for you? For example, you've just graduated, you've been working hard applying for jobs, and you receive notice that you've been short-listed for an interview with a highly desirable company. Or you've been trying to have a baby, and finally a pregnancy test comes back positive. Or you've moved into a new area and tried connecting with your neighbors; after several initiatives, you get an invitation to a neighborhood social gathering. Or, after a long dry spell, you finally play your best round of golf ever. Going back to our definition of happiness, you can see that in all these examples you not only felt pleasure, but also made progress toward accomplishing some valued goal because of your own effort. Taking responsibility, exercising personal control (i.e., putting forth active effort), and making significant gains in working on a valued goal are important aspects of happiness and joy.

To understand your personal pursuit of happiness, reflect on your past experiences of feeling significant positive emotion. They may be related to accomplishments at work or school, in relationships, or with your family; they could be connected with some sporting activity, hobby, vacation, or recreational pursuit. Was there an important life goal or value involved in one of your recent happy experiences? Was your joy associated with making progress toward the goal or with living according to the value? Was there a feeling that you accomplished something because of your own efforts? One of my happiest times was the birth of our older daughter. I remember leaving the hospital the night of her birth, kicking my heels in the air, and singing my favorite tune (no one was around to witness this!). For me, it had all the elements of happiness. In particular, it accomplished several valued goals: My wife and the baby were healthy; the event marked the beginning of our family; and the anxieties and uncertainties associated with pregnancy were ended.

If you're having trouble remembering happy experiences, you could ask a family member or close friend for some help. Likewise, if your list of happy experiences seems short, the problem may be that you haven't paid sufficient attention to your happy experiences. Taking some time to reflect on your happy moments is important, because you may have focused so much on sadness that you've forgotten what happiness is like. Also, it's good to remind yourself that you are capable of happiness. If you created happiness in the past, there is definitely hope for the future! I'll return to this topic later, when the first mood enhancement strategy is discussed.

> Reflect on past memories of happiness. Have you forgotten that you once felt happiness and joy in your life?

Before I present the mood enhancement strategies, it's important to place this discussion of happiness within the context of life satisfaction and well-being more generally—a context that has been referred to as *positive psychology*. Martin Seligman, a professor of psychology at the University of Pennsylvania, is one of the foremost experts on positive psychology and author of the book *Flourish*. He describes five elements of a worthwhile life or a sense of well-being:[2]

- *Positive emotion*—the experience of positive affect, such as happiness, joy, pride, comfort, or interest.
- *Engagement*—becoming completely absorbed in an activity, to the point where you feel as if time stops and you've lost self-consciousness.
- *Meaning*—belonging to and serving something bigger than yourself (e.g., religious groups, political parties, community organizations, nonprofits).
- *Accomplishment*—the pursuit of success, achievement, and mastery for their own sakes, rather than simply as a means to acquire more money or status.
- *Positive relationships*—the ability to give and receive love in social relationships, and to pursue positive, caring relationships with others for their own sakes.

Seligman sets up a hierarchy of sorts when it comes to positive functioning. *Happiness* is characterized by positive emotion, engagement, and meaning—three of the five elements of a worthwhile life. Happiness is central to *well-being*, but the latter is a much bigger concept. Numerous studies have shown that a greater sense of well-being is associated with better physical health; resilience against life's adversities; lower rates of depression and anxiety; better family and couple relationships; and higher work performance and career success. So these are further reasons for working on happiness and well-being: Not only will you feel better, but you'll have a better life more generally.

Another reason for working on positive emotion is that it will help reduce your problem with depressed mood. Most self-help books deal with sadness and happiness separately; you will find books on overcoming depression and others on living the happy life, but most often the two are not considered under the same title. However, I believe it is important to consider both sides of the fence: reducing negative mood and enhancing positive emotion. Seligman has stated this succinctly in *Flourish*:

> The skills of enjoying positive emotion, being engaged with the people you care about, having meaning in life, achieving your work goals, and maintaining good relationships are entirely different from the skills of not being depressed, not being anxious, and not being angry. (p. 182)

In the spirit of this distinction, you will notice that I refer to the exercises in this chapter as *mood enhancement* rather than *mood repair* strategies. (I also use just "Strategy" instead of "Repair Strategy" in the strategy numbers for this chapter, although the numbers are continuous with those for the earlier mood repair strategies.)

There are several other reasons for wanting to enhance positive emotion in its own right. Several years ago, researchers reviewed a large number of studies on the benefits of frequent positive emotion.[3] Their conclusion was that happy people tend to be more successful and flourishing. Even though happy people experience occasional periods of unhappiness, and they can react negatively to bad events, they tend to maintain a positive mood state more often than not. Psychologist Sonja Lyubomirsky and colleagues reported that positive affect (i.e., happiness) is moderately associated with life satisfaction, and the majority of happy people report that they feel happy at least half of the time. In regard to tangible outcomes, they concluded that happy people are more likely to be high performers at work, to earn higher incomes, to be more engaged in their communities, to have better social relationships (including marriages), to have better physical and mental health, and to live longer.[3] Moreover, happiness appears to play a causal role in bringing about these positive outcomes. Given all of the benefits associated with happiness, who would not want to work on increasing daily positive emotion, regardless of vulnerability to the blues?

Spend time on positive mood enhancement if you want to . . .

- feel more happiness in your life.
- reduce your tendency to become depressed.
- be stronger in response to life's problems and difficulties.
- have better physical health, as well as better family and social relations.
- be more productive and successful in your career.
- live longer.

➤ Strategy 75: Keep a Happiness Diary

It may be human nature to notice the negative things that happen to us more quickly and efficiently than the positive things. Situations involving loss, failure, and danger threaten our survival, whereas success, achievement, and mastery experiences have much less immediate effects. If you find yourself walking alone late at night in a sketchy part of the city, it's probably a lot more adaptive to be having fearful thoughts focused on anticipating danger than more positive, optimistic thoughts of safety and comfort. Of course, not that much of daily life is taken up with dangerous situations (for most middle- and upper-income North Americans), and yet the negativity bias continues to operate. What this means is that a lot of really good things—some small ones, but even the larger ones—may go relatively unnoticed.

Earlier in the chapter, I have suggested that you reflect back on past experiences of happiness. Did you find it hard to remember happy moments in your life? Is this because nothing good has happened in your life, or is it because a negativity bias is operating and you don't really pay attention to positive experiences? If you don't process these experiences, they become quickly forgotten, replaced by memories of the negative things. Naturally, if you are tuned in to the negative and missing the positive, your mood level will tend to match your attentional bias. So the first step toward greater happiness is learning to catch the good things that are happening on a daily basis.

> **Start tracking daily experiences of joy and happiness.**

TOOL FINDER The early chapters in this book have discussed the fact that those frequently stuck in the blues may have a particularly strong negativity bias. You may have already practiced noticing your experience more objectively when you monitored your hourly emotions in Chapter 2, or when you recorded your negative automatic thoughts in Chapter 4. All of the exercises early in the book provide good practice for reacquainting yourself with what your real experience feels like.

STRATEGY 75 INSTRUCTIONS

1. **To get started with your Happiness Diary, review the entries you made in the daily diaries you completed in Chapters 2 (Repair Strategy 2) and 5 (Repair Strategy 17).** Note the experiences or activities that were associated with high ratings of enjoyment or times of the day when you felt a higher level of happiness. Over the next 2 weeks, pay particular attention to the times during the day when you feel more positive or when you engage in high-enjoyment activities. Become more conscious of your happiness level during these times, and enter the experiences in your Happiness Diary. You can use the partial form on the facing page to create your Happiness Diary, or you can print out the complete form from *www. guilford.com/clark7-forms*.

2. **At the end of each day, take a few minutes to review the positive experiences you recorded in your Happiness Diary. Do you see any patterns—any recurrences in the things that made you feel some degree of joy or happiness?** Make

Happiness Diary

Briefly describe positive experience, activity, event	Level of positive feeling (0–10)	Consequences or impact of positive experience on your mood, behavior, and/or relations with others

sure you've written down specific details of each event and noted why it made you feel so good, so you can use this information to genuinely reexperience past moments of happiness. Also make sure you've written down the little things that caused even a slight bump in the positive direction for your mood, as well as the bigger events that made you feel really happy. Of course, don't feel that your diary has to be exhaustive. You don't need to record everything, but you should include two or three things each day that caused an increase in positive mood.

3. **Take time to truly "savor" the positive experiences in each day, so hold on to your thoughts about the happiness experience for a minute or two.** The following are some questions you can ask about your "happiness entries" in order to recall the positive experiences more fully.

> "What happened in this situation that caused me to feel happy?"
>
> "How did I react in this situation? What part did I play in bringing about this positive outcome?"
>
> "Did anyone say anything to me, or respond to me in a way, that made me feel valued, wanted, or appreciated? Were my efforts acknowledged in some way?"
>
> "What important goal or value was affirmed in this situation?"

Recall that one of the problems with feeling depressed is that you are not paying attention to positive daily experiences. The Happiness Diary improves attention to the positive by encouraging you to spend time reflecting on the positive experiences in your day. More time in reflection will improve your memory for the positive. In turn, you can use your improved memory for positive experiences to enhance your mood, because a more vivid recall of good things from the past should boost your mood in the positive direction. This will be helpful in shifting you from a negative to a more positive perspective.

Here are two examples of hypothetical Happiness Diary entries.

> Today, April 26, 2013, I met with [student's name], and out of the blue she told me that a skills course she took from me last year was the most helpful course she's taken in graduate school for providing her with critical therapy skills needed to treat people with psychological problems. I instantly felt a surge of positive emotion that was a combination of surprise, gratitude, and pride. It made me feel that all the work I've put into preparing my graduate courses was making a difference, and that at least some students were appreciating my teaching efforts. It made me feel valued as a teacher, which is an important part of how I define my personal career success.

> On August 28, 2010, my youngest daughter, who was 19 years old at the time, took me to a Boston Red Sox game at Fenway Park as a birthday gift. Although she is a university student with limited income, she paid all the expenses. It was one of the most enjoyable days of my life, even though I'm not a strong baseball fan. What made this so special was the effort and thoughtfulness she put into the gift and the fact that she wanted to spend a Saturday afternoon with her father. This was important to me because I value family relationships, and it confirmed that I was loved and that over the years we have together built a good father–daughter relationship.

Although these two examples involved a sense of gratitude for acts of kindness extended toward me, your Happiness Diary entries could just as easily involve something you've accomplished (e.g., completing a difficult project, getting a promotion, doing a best time run, etc.), a new relationship, or just a happy feeling because of the circumstances of the moment.

Use Strategy 75 to lift your mood state by . . .

- countering your tendency to attend to and remember negative things.
- helping instill a sense of gratitude for the good things in your life.
- creating more experiences of feeling happy or joyful, because of being intentional about taking notice of the positives in your daily life.
- encouraging a positive or more optimistic mindset throughout the day.

⟫⟫⟫➡ Strategy ⑦⑥: Nurture Gratitude in Your Life

Try to remember the last time someone showed kindness toward you. It could have been something quite significant (such as a coworker's taking your shift so you could attend your child's school concert) or something relatively minor (like a fellow shopper's letting you jump ahead in a long line because you seemed particularly rushed). How did that act of kindness make you feel? No doubt you experienced a spike in positive emotion that, although brief, caused a positive change in how you felt. And if you expressed gratitude for the kindness of the other person, you would have felt even better. Psychologists have begun to study gratitude, because it turns out that being thankful or having gratitude has a considerable impact on life satisfaction and well-being.

But first let's be clear about what we mean by *gratitude*. Researchers Robert Emmons and Michael McCullough[4] define gratitude as a positive emotion characterized by *thankfulness*, or "the perception of a positive personal outcome, not necessarily deserved or earned, that is due to the actions of another person" (p. 377). In fact, most of the research on gratitude has focused on this idea of a benefactor's providing a benefit to a beneficiary. For example, I (the benefactor) give you (the beneficiary) my seat on the bus (a benefit). The general public, on the other hand, tends to think of gratitude more broadly as expressing appreciation for what is valuable and meaningful in one's life (e.g., feeling gratitude for living in a free, democratic society). For the purposes of this exercise, we'll restrict ourselves to the narrower definition of gratitude, which refers to the kind actions of others.

There is mounting evidence that gratitude not only broadens thought and behavior, but builds enduring personal resources. A greater sense of gratitude or thankfulness is associated with a higher level of life satisfaction, more optimism, higher levels of positive affect and lower levels of negative affect, better health behavior (e.g., more time spent exercising, better sleep), a greater sense of connectedness with others, and fewer depressive symptoms.[5] At least some of these positive effects are due to individuals' being able to understand negative experiences from a more positive perspective (e.g., "I did poorly on the exam, but I am grateful that Julie shared her lecture notes with me because they helped me at least pass "). These positive effects are apparent whether gratitude is measured as a personality trait (i.e., being a thankful person) or is manipulated in an experimental design (i.e., inducing high or low levels of gratitude). This suggests that you can work on increasing the level of gratitude in your daily living, which in turn will have beneficial effects on mood and general well-being. Interestingly, the opposite of gratitude—heightened envy or a focus on daily hassles—may have a negative effect on well-being.

> Grateful people are happier, better adjusted, and less depressed.

Use Strategy 76 when you . . .

- are critical of others, tending to focus on their faults and shortcomings.

- are highly self-focused on negative experiences.

- struggle with a pessimistic, even cynical, outlook on life.

- believe people are basically selfish and uncaring, especially toward you.

STRATEGY 76 INSTRUCTIONS

There are several things you can do to nurture the positive emotion of gratitude in your life.

1. **Keep a gratitude journal.** One of the best ways to increase your sense of gratitude is to keep a gratitude journal in which you make entries at the end of each day. Write down anything that happened to you today for which you are grateful or thankful. Most of these entries will involve acts of kindness toward you by others at work, at home, or in your community. You can, however, broaden the exercise to include anything for which you are thankful, such as clean air to breathe, sunshine, or lighter traffic. As you do this exercise, truly think about the blessings in your life, and don't just jot down a few things as if you were making a grocery list. If someone has treated you kindly, think about the person and what his/her action means about the person and about you. Make sure you spend a few minutes savoring these acts of goodness in your life. This exercise will overlap with keeping the Happiness Diary. Many of your happy events will also involve gratitude, as did my two examples in Strategy 75. It is okay to do these exercises together; it's just that a gratitude journal is a little more focused on your expression of thankfulness and a little less focused on your level of happiness.

2. **Practice gratitude-focused meditation.** Spend 15–20 minutes several times a week in mindfulness meditation. After attaining a meditative state through focus on your breath and body scanning, gently shift your attention to something in your life that fills you with a deep sense of appreciation. Most often this will involve a spouse/partner, parent, other family member, or very close friend with whom you have strong, loving connections and who has shown significant loving care toward you. Notice that in gratitude-focused meditation you will be concentrating on the truly significant acts of kindness, which engender a deep sense of gratitude. Since gratitude-focused meditation should be practiced repeatedly, you will want several examples of loving kindness to use in your meditation practice.

TOOL FINDER See Chapter 7 for more detailed instructions on meditation. This exercise is similar to meditative self-compassion (see Chapter 11, Repair Strategy 48). The difference is that in gratitude-focused meditation, you focus your attention on heartfelt thankfulness for the good that you have received in this life.

3. **Create a gratitude testimonial.** Another way to develop gratitude is to write and then deliver a gratitude letter to a person you never properly thanked for a previous act of kindness.[2] In one page, describe in some detail what the person did for you and how it positively affected your life. After composing the letter, you could meet with the benefactor (if this is possible) and slowly read the testimonial, giving time for each of you to digest the contents. Obviously, this exercise should be done very selectively and only with individuals who have had a profound impact on your life.

4. **Engage in acts of graciousness.** There is a close relationship between more kindness and more gratitude: Kinder people experience more happiness and gratitude in their daily lives. Thus one way to increase gratitude might be to practice more kindness and generosity toward others. You can do this intentionally by keeping track of the number of kind acts you perform on a daily basis. The purpose of this exercise is not to engage in self-congratulatory behavior, but simply to raise your level of conscious awareness of being kind.

> **Intentionally increase acts of kindness to heighten gratitude.**

TOOL FINDER This exercise has been covered in greater detail in Chapter 11 (Repair Strategy 50).

⟫⟫⟫➤ Strategy **77**: Know Your Strengths

Have you ever met with a financial advisor to go over your financial portfolio? How useful would it be if the advisor focused only on your debts and losses, and completely ignored your income and assets? Not only would it be discouraging, but it would be entirely useless for formulating a wealth management plan. And yet the reality is that millions of people take such a negatively skewed approach when they engage in any self-evaluation. We seem to have a natural tendency to readily acknowledge personal weaknesses and failures, while ignoring our strengths and talents. Like getting bad financial advice, living life with a negative perspective on yourself is not conducive to positive emotion and well-being. Recognizing the strengths in your character is considered an important pathway to life satisfaction and increased happiness.

Use Strategy 77 when you . . .

- are stuck in self-criticism and excessive negativity.
- can't see anything good or positive about yourself.
- feel embarrassed and reject or minimize recognition, compliments, or praise from others.

STRATEGY 77 INSTRUCTIONS

1. **Use the Personal Positive Characteristics Record template on the facing page to begin a systematic examination of your personal strengths or characteristics.** A more detailed Personal Positive Characteristics Record—which includes more probing questions for each domain, plus instructions on how to complete the record—can be downloaded from *www.guilford.com/clark7-forms*, or you can photocopy the basic template here. The ability to recognize your good qualities is related to increased happiness, so reflecting on your strengths will be well worth the investment in time. If you are having trouble thinking about your strengths in these various life domains, ask a close friend or family member to help you complete the Personal Positive Characteristics Record. It is likely that you've never thought about your strengths and abilities in these different areas of your life. For example, let's consider the Relationships domain. Think about the various relationships in your life and how you tend to deal with people. You might conclude that these are your strengths: You can understand other people; you really do care for the welfare of others; you're emotionally sensitive to people's needs; and you do go out of your way to show kindness to others. So these would be the strengths you would write down in the third column of the Personal Positive Characteristics Record. Then you would go back to the second column and rate your level of success in the relationship domain on the 0–5 scale there, where 0 = no success and 5 = completely successful. It is likely that no one can be rated as a 0 or a 5 in any domain, but you should notice varying levels of success as you consider these various facets of your life. Remember the goal of this exercise is not to highlight areas that need improvement, but rather to help you appreciate your strengths and to see that you are doing well in some areas of your life.

Personal Positive Characteristics Record

Life domains	Rate level of success (0–5)	Give examples of personal strengths associated with this domain
A. Relationships What are your strengths in how you relate to your partner, children, parents, other family, friends, even strangers?		
B. Achievement What are your strengths in how you approach work, learning, being productive?		
C. Health and well-being What are your strengths in self-care?		
D. Leisure and recreation What are your strengths in pursuing leisure, recreation, having fun?		
E. Civic duty and responsibility What are your strengths in duty and commitment to country, state/province, and community life?		
F. Spirituality What are your strengths in nurturing a sense of spirituality—the transcendence in your life?		

An alternative approach to strengths assessment has been developed by Martin Seligman. He proposes 24 character strengths, which he clusters into five value domains: wisdom and knowledge; courage, humanity, and love; justice; temperance; and transcendence or spirituality.[2] For further information on Seligman's strengths assessment, see the University of Pennsylvania Positive Psychology website (*www.authentichappiness.sas.upenn.edu*). It is well worth the time to register on this website and take the Brief Strengths Test.

2. **Now look back over the Personal Positive Characteristics Record you completed, especially the examples you listed in the third column.** How did you do in listing examples of your strengths? If you had difficulty, think about examples of your strengths when it comes to specific aspects of each life domain. What are some of the things you do best? Once these have been identified, ask yourself why you excel in these areas. This is another way to identify your character strengths. For example, one of my friends is very well liked and so has many male friends, which is quite unusual for a middle-aged Canadian man. The qualities he brings to these friendships are kindness, generosity, understanding, tolerance, and humility. These are his character strengths, and so others like to be around him. I'm not sure my friend actually recognizes his character strengths, but all he has to do is to examine his daily activities to understand himself better.

> The tasks you do best provide clues to your character strengths.

3. **Once you know your character strengths, you will need to capitalize on them for this knowledge to have any effect on positive mood.** Each day, take one of your character strengths and think about the different ways you express that strength in your daily living. Then consider how you can capitalize on the strength in your work, family life, and relationships with others. For example, let's say you've identified a desire to learn as one of your character strengths under the Achievement domain. You could decide to start a new hobby, like investigating your genealogy or learning woodworking, which would express this desire. If you have a strong sense of citizenship as indicated in the Civic Duty and Responsibility domain, you could join some community or civic initiatives. You should experience a boost in positive emotions as you engage in activities that build on your character strengths.

➤➤➤ Strategy ⑦⑧: Strive for the 3:1 Rule

As noted in Chapter 2, the average person experiences longer and more frequent positive than negative daily moods. But is there a ratio of positive to negative mood that is optimally related to happiness and life satisfaction? And what about the positive and negative thoughts associated with our mood states? Is there an optimal ratio of positive to negative thoughts, too?

You may recall from the first chapter that a mild positive mood state character-izes normal daily living, except for persons struggling with frequent depressed mood. Having a positivity bias is quite adaptive, because positive emotions broaden thoughts and actions and encourage exploration, growth, flexibility, and nurturance over the long term.[6] To maintain a mildly positive state, an individual would have to experi-ence more positive than negative thoughts and feelings. However, if we go beyond simple ordinary existence and ask about optimal living or flourishing, how many posi-tive thoughts and emotions are necessary? In terms of emotional functioning, it turns out that a positivity ratio of at least 3:1—three positive emotions to one negative—is needed to exhibit flourishing.[6] In the realm of cognitions, at least four or possibly five positive thoughts for every negative are needed to attain an optimal level of happiness and well-being.[7] Individuals who experience more negative than positive thoughts are at greatest risk for low self-esteem and depressive mood, but even dropping below the 3:1 ratio of positive to negative feelings can be associated with languishing—not feel-ing depressed, but feeling that life is hollow or empty.[6] The bottom line is that reduc-ing negative thinking is critical for repairing depressed mood (see Chapter 4), but that boosting positive thinking and experiences is critical for happiness and well-being.

Most of us can be much more intentional about boosting both positive emotions and positive thinking in our daily lives. How much time do you spend thinking about your accomplishments, pleasant experiences, compliments, positive feedback, and the like, relative to pondering your failures, disappointments, and criticisms? How much of your day is spent pursuing pleasant, positive experiences as opposed to dealing with stress and adversity? To be sure, none of us can ignore the problems and negative stuff that happens in our lives. To live in denial or avoidance of our problems (see Chapter 13) is unhelpful and even harmful. But the question here is one of relative emphasis. To what extent are you minimizing or neglecting positive thoughts, feelings, and experiences, to the detriment of your own happiness and sense of well-being? Is it not time to intention-ally recalibrate your emotional thermostat, so that you find yourself on the upper side of the positivity divide?

Use Strategy 78 when you . . .

- experience more negative than positive thoughts and feelings in your daily living.

- experience repeated and/or persistent negative mood.

- believe you're incapable of positive thoughts or feelings.

STRATEGY 78 INSTRUCTIONS

1. **At the end of each day, take a few minutes to review your daily experiences. Take note of positive experiences, your accomplishments, and any compliments from others.** Refer back to your Happiness Diary for reminders if you have used Strategy 75.

2. **Ponder how you contributed to each positive experience or accomplishment. Above all, practice the art of giving yourself credit when credit is due.**

3. **Use your knowledge of how your own initiative contributed to positive experiences to increase your positive–negative emotions ratio to at least 3:1.** Engaging in positive self-talk is not an arrogant act of self-promotion. Instead, your goal is to recognize the good within you at the same time as you maintain a realistic view of life experiences and circumstances. If it helps, think about what you would say to a friend who did the same thing or had the same experience. Would you not participate in the friend's good news—maybe by pointing out his/her positive contribution to bringing about the experience (e.g., "I'm so pleased you got the promotion! You've been so productive in your work that you certainly deserved the recognition")? The important point is to learn to talk nicely to yourself—to be as positive with yourself as you would be with close friends and family members. Remember, we all need to follow the 3:1 rule to feel happy and fulfilled.

⯈⯈⯈⯈ Strategy 79: Practice the Art of Being Just Satisfied

Not everything we do is a matter of life or death. Some tasks are much more important than others, and so we all have to prioritize. We should devote a lot more time and effort to tasks that are high in personal value, and less time and resources to activities that matter little to our overall well-being. But the management of our time and effort is not an exact science, and so it is easy to overdo things (see the "Less Is Best" sidebar on the facing page).

Of course, the more important a task or decision is for your general well-being, the greater the need will be to move from a satisfying approach to a maximizing orientation (as described in the sidebar). Taking a "good enough" approach to deciding which lawn care company to employ to cut your grass makes a lot of sense, whereas a maximizing perspective is needed in deciding to take a new job in a different city. However, the point is that often people rob themselves of happiness and well-being by taking everything too seriously and being unable to accept that many things in life are not that important—that a satisfactory outcome is often "good enough." Doing "less

less is best

Over 50 years ago, Herbert Simon at the Carnegie Institute of Technology argued that organisms learn and make choices based on pursuing a path that leads to satisfaction at some threshold of acceptability, rather than an ideal path of maximizing that would result in some optimal adaptation.[8] Much later, Barry Schwartz and colleagues at Swarthmore College extended Simon's theory, arguing that too many decision-making options can have negative effects on well-being, and that people differ in whether they seek the maximum or can be satisfied with less than the best.[9] In other words, some people, called *maximizers* by Schwartz et al., tend to search for the very best (if not perfect) solution when making a decision. Because of this, they try to consider as many options as possible—but this creates a problem for them, because the more options they review, the less likely they are to find the optimal solution. People who can live with less than the best seek solutions that simply meet a threshold of acceptability or satisfaction, since their criterion is "good enough." Having more options is not a problem for these more easily satisfied persons, since they can simply ignore the alternatives.

> Making satisfactory decisions, rather than insisting on the absolute best, is associated with greater happiness and well-being.

Schwartz and colleagues have made a compelling argument that maximizing may have negative effects on well-being, whereas being satisfied may be the more positive approach. They developed a Maximization Scale, with high scores reflecting a combination of perfectionism, indecision, and need to consider a wide array of options. In a series of studies, they found that maximizers had more regrets and were more perfectionistic and depressed, whereas people who operated from a satisfaction perspective were more optimistic, more satisfied with life, happier, and had higher self-esteem.[9] The advantage of having satisfaction or acceptability (i.e., "good enough") as your criterion is that decision making takes less time and effort; it's psychologically less taxing, so making decisions is quicker. People who are guided by satisfaction are less indecisive, feel better about their choices, and have fewer regrets than maximizers.[9] As a result, people who practice the "art of achieving a grade of satisfactory," as indicated by lower scores on the Maximization Scale, are happier and have higher life satisfaction.

than the best" can play an important role in creating a more contented, happier daily life.

If you are a maximizer, then learning to experience the state of "just satisfied" versus "my very best" may be important to increasing your level of daily happiness. However, you may find it difficult to shift to a "less than best" mentality. You can use the following interventions to help reshape your focus.

Use Strategy 79 when you . . .

- have perfectionistic tendencies.
- lack confidence in decision making.
- experience doubts or regrets toward your decisions.
- struggle with procrastination or other types of avoidance.
- "overthink" and/or overcontrol personal situations, tasks, and responsibilities.

STRATEGY 79 INSTRUCTIONS

1. **Take a close look at friends or work colleagues who appear to take a more "laid-back" approach to life.** What do you think of their standards? Are they selective in where they apply their "just satisfied" criteria? Do you notice any positive or negative consequences with their more relaxed personal standards? You might want to write down your observations and think about whether they might be usefully applied in your life.

   Gerry was always stressed out and unhappy at work. She felt insecure as the most recent hire in a large law firm. Everything she did, from answering correspondence to responding to office emails, she did to the best of her ability. However, she noticed that her staff colleagues took a much more relaxed approach. They seemed less stressed and actually happier at work. As Gerry took a closer look at their work habits, she noticed that they spent little time editing their internal office emails, which were voluminous and time-consuming. They would get the job done, but were not too concerned about grammar or typos. Gerry realized that she needed to adopt their standard when it came to internal emails; a "good enough" standard was sufficient. She needed to stop torturing herself with "over the top" email standards. Gerry began to look around at other standards that she might be able to relax so that she could feel more enjoyment at work.

2. **After observing others, become more self-focused in how you work and relate to others.** Why not keep a "good enough" journal over the next 2–3 weeks?

Each day, write down some experiences that were not your best but were "good enough." These could be tasks you have accomplished or decisions that you have taken on various issues. For example, you didn't take the quickest way to work this morning, but it was OK; it took a little longer, but it was "good enough." You wanted to get 40 minutes of exercise this morning, but you ended up with 30 minutes, and that was "good enough" for today. You went to the grocery store, but you didn't sit down beforehand and figure out the list and meal plan for the next several days. Instead, you went and spontaneously picked up a few items. It wasn't the most economical or efficient way to do grocery shopping, because you'll probably have to go back in a couple of days and pick up more items, but it was satisfactory for today. In our highly competitive society, we often lose perspective, thinking we have to do our very best at every decision and activity. The reality is that striving for an A+ in everything we do is bad for our mental health; a B, or even a C+, is often sufficient and associated with a better sense of well-being.

3. **Finally, work on making some changes to your personal standards.** We all make a multitude of decisions throughout the day. Take a look at how you make decisions and ask yourself whether you are overdoing it—expending far too much time and effort searching all the options in an attempt to make the very best decisions. But is that really necessary? Are you overestimating the significance and value of some decisions? Would the "good enough" rule apply? Practice decision making based on the "good enough" criterion, and then make note of the consequences. Were you justified in taking a satisfactory rather than a maximizing perspective on this decision? Each time you make a satisfactory decision and notice the consequences, you are strengthening your ability to live in the state of satisfaction—an important pathway to happiness and well-being.

►►►► Strategy ⑧⓪: Enrich your Interpersonal Relations

The quality of our social relationships has a profound impact on whether we are happy and satisfied. Just as loneliness, social isolation, interpersonal conflict, and rejection can lead to discouragement and despair, so can healthy and harmonious relationships contribute to happiness and greater life satisfaction. A specific focus on active, constructive responding is a key communication strategy for turning good relationships into excellent ones—the types of enhanced relationship that can boost happiness and life satisfaction.[2] Chapter 10 has focused on overcoming social isolation or difficult relationships to repair negative mood, whereas here we are talking about enriching ordinary relationships in order to boost positive mood states.

TOOL FINDER The eight strategies presented in Chapter 10 can also be used to enhance your social life and encourage positive emotion and happiness.

An important way to enrich relationships is to practice active, constructive responding: listening carefully when valued friends or family members tell you about good things that have happened in their lives. When you show interest, ask questions about their experiences; in essence, you are asking them to relive the experiences for you. Notice that the focus is on listening intently to the positive experiences in other people's lives. It's on complimenting them, expressing genuine pleasure in their accomplishment or good fortune. For illustrative purposes, my daughter recently got accepted into her top choice for graduate school. Below, I present a healthy way and several unhealthy ways I could have responded to her good news.

> **The way we respond to the good news of loved ones affects the health of our relationships.**

Active Healthy Response

"Christina, that's great news! Well done. What did the acceptance letter say? How did you feel before opening it and then after reading the first line? Who did you tell about it, and what did they say? I am so proud of you. This is a tremendous accomplishment, and you really deserved to be accepted. You've worked hard to get to this point, and your future looks so bright and exciting. What do you plan to do next? What are your thoughts about getting ready for graduate school? Let's go out and celebrate this great news."

Active Negative Response

"I'm really surprised that you got accepted. Sounds like a lot of work. Are you up for the challenge? You'll have to study hard and work long hours; you've always had trouble with your motivation in the past. Aren't you afraid of moving to a strange city by yourself? How will you ever manage on your own?"

Passive Constructive Response

"Great news! I'm so happy for you." [I then go back to answering my email correspondence, so I am failing to validate her positive experience.]

Passive Negative Response

"I'm so busy at work; I don't know how I'll get all my work done." [I basically ignore my daughter when she enters the room, and I don't even give her a chance to share her good news.]

There is evidence that responding to the positive experiences of our intimate partners with active and constructive responses is a significant predictor of relationship well-being, at least over the short term.[10] People we are close to often tell us their good news, their accomplishments and victories. How we respond to their good news plays an important role in whether our relationships with them are enriched or starved. If you want to avoid impoverished connections with loved ones, you need to learn how to celebrate their good news with them.

STRATEGY 80 INSTRUCTIONS

1. **A little soul-searching can be helpful. Take a close look at how you interact with your loved ones, and ask yourself the following questions:**

   "How much genuine interest do I have in the lives of my spouse/partner, family members, and friends?"

   "Do I know how to celebrate their successes and good news?"

   "How often do I ask them questions about their experiences, or what is happening in their daily lives?"

   "How well do I show sensitivity, empathy, and real understanding for their feelings?"

   "Can I truly listen to them, or do I talk more about myself?"

   "Can I accept their positive experiences without social comparison—without a sense of jealousy or envy for their good fortune?"

   The extent to which you can truly connect with your loved ones, in good times as well as bad, will determine the richness of your relationships. Building strong, healthy relationships depends on a capacity to give and receive love and care, which in turn is an important determinant of happiness and well-being.

2. **Initiate conversations with family or friends, making sure to ask about any good news or developments in their lives.** When having a conversation with people

you know, make sure to ask them about anything good that has happened to them lately. If you've heard good news, ask further questions showing genuine interest in their success or good fortune. Practice the active listening skills discussed previously.

3. **If you use social media, respond to the good news that friends post on Facebook or Twitter.** Many people report their every move on social media, and this is especially true when it involves some positive development in their lives. Responding to positive postings on Facebook, Twitter, Instagram, and the like is a great way to show active response to family, friends, and coworkers. It can help you develop an attitude of response and caring toward others.

4. **Intentionally practice active listening in daily casual conversation.** Whether at work, home, or some other social context, practice active listening in your interaction with others. You could even train yourself to be a better listener by seeing if you can write down the main points of what a person said to you in an earlier conversation. Were you tracking what the person was talking about, or were you thinking about something else that diverted your attention away from the conversation? Active, constructive listening is just that: listening and remembering.

Thriving in the 21st Century

This chapter has shifted our focus of attention from strategies for reducing negative mood to ones that emphasize growth, vitality, and positive emotion. Thriving in the 21st century depends more than ever on positive health and well-being. To *thrive* or *flourish* means to live within the bounds of goodness, nurturance, growth, and resilience.[6] Positive mental health involves the experience of happiness, purposeful engagement in life activities, a sense of meaning, healthy relationships, and perceived accomplishment. It also involves exhibiting resilience in the face of adversity, and living a life that balances adaptive response to challenges and difficulties with frequent experiences of joy and contentment. Living a good life means more than the absence of negative emotion, if that were even possible; it also includes enrichment of positive emotion and well-being. Thriving in the present age is particularly challenging, since our postmodern era is a crucible for negative emotion. Negative mood repair is one approach to improving your present life, but the other side of the coin is to accentuate positive feelings through mood enhancement strategies. The mood work described in this chapter plays a critical role in the development of healthy emotional well-being.

Although genetics and personality do have a strong influence on our emotional makeup, the good news is that everyone experiences positive mood or happiness at least some of the time. As noted previously, the majority of people report relatively high levels of general satisfaction with life, and in the typical day they experience more happiness than sadness, thereby creating what is called the *positivity offset* (see Chapter 1 for discussion). Of course, differences exist among individuals in the frequency, intensity, and duration of their moments of happiness. But everyone has at least some experience of happiness to start with; we all have a foundation to build on. We can start with the positive experiences we already have and work on expanding the quantity and quality of happiness in our daily lives.

The single most important factor in life satisfaction is the frequency of positive emotion. I am convinced that you will find mood enhancement activities well worth the time and effort. They will enrich your quality of life by allowing you to harness your potential for greater happiness in daily living, and they will produce more life satisfaction and general well-being than will an incessant preoccupation with success, status, and wealth accumulation. Indeed, these latter pursuits have been linked to increased anxiety, insecurity, jealousy, and despair. So what's stopping you from embracing a more holistic, positive approach to your emotional well-being?

15 take the long view

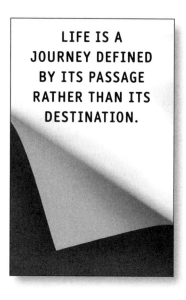

LIFE IS A JOURNEY DEFINED BY ITS PASSAGE RATHER THAN ITS DESTINATION.

In years gone by, workhorse teams were harnessed so that their massive strength could be channeled into productive work like plowing fields or harvesting crops—work that was critical to the survival of our forebears. This is an apt analogy for the work of emotion regulation. In Chapter 1, I have talked about the "joy of sadness"—the fact that negative emotions are not only normal, but also beneficial. We need periods of feeling blue to reflect on our circumstances and plan for the future. Like a workhorse, however, this mood state needs to be harnessed to be used productively. When our periods of sadness become too intense or prolonged, they can cause significant distress and interfere with our ability to function. Daily bouts of low mood can rob us of life satisfaction and well-being. To avoid such a negative impact, we must work with our sadness, turning it into a contributor to life adjustment rather than a detriment to well-being.

The negative mood repair and positive mood enhancement strategies presented in this book are intended to help you harness your negativity—to turn the times of feeling down and discouraged into more productive reflection, planning, and immediate action. If handled properly, these periods can mobilize you to deal effectively with the problems and difficulties of daily living. Mood repair can be used to experience sadness in a healthy rather than an unhealthy fashion. This final chapter covers three topics that are important for maintaining a positive approach to negative mood:

- The signs that sadness has become clinical depression, meaning that the self-help approach to negative mood may be insufficient and professional consultation may be advisable.
- Obstacles or difficulties that could hinder the effectiveness of mood repair.
- The influence of personal life goals, values, and meaning on quality of life and emotional well-being.

Deciding When to Seek Professional Help

The mood repair strategies presented in this book can be helpful for the full range of depressed mood, from mild occasional sadness to more prolonged states of despair where you may not even have sufficient energy to get out of bed. However, the more intense and prolonged your depressed feelings are, the more difficult it becomes to repair mood on your own. When your negative mood state approaches the range of a clinical disorder, you will have major struggles with lack of motivation, fatigue, and loss of interest. Even basic tasks of daily living take a great deal of effort, and little or no energy is left for tasks like the mood repair exercises described in this book.

If you feel this depleted, it is time to consult a mental health professional—a psychiatrist, psychologist, social worker, or other mental health therapist. Since many of the strategies in this book are derived from treatments for depression, your mental health therapist will probably draw on some of these mood repair strategies in her treatment plan. In fact you and your therapist may decide to use *The Mood Repair Toolkit* as a supplementary resource for your therapy. Whatever the case, one of the most obvious signs of the need to seek professional help is when you have little motivation to engage in mood repair on your own.

> When your motivation is too low to engage in mood repair, it's time to seek professional help.

Lack of motivation isn't the only sign that you might need professional help. If your depressed mood is persistent, day after day, with little relief, then it is probably time to consider treatment. Likewise, if you start experiencing a lot of symptoms that are making it hard to function (in addition to feeling down and discouraged), you may qualify for a diagnosis of clinical depression and should seek treatment from a qualified mental health professional. Only a professional can make a reliable diagnosis, but in general you may start to feel physically, mentally, and emotionally impaired, and these feelings may go on for days. Maybe you dread getting out of bed and then drag yourself around all day, no longer interested in your usual activities or the special events that usually give you pleasure. Have your eating and sleeping habits changed—you don't even relish your favorite foods, and you either can't seem to get enough sleep or can't get to sleep at all? Are you watching projects languish and deadlines pass because you can't muster the mental focus to get things done or the physical energy to follow through? Do you find yourself pacing restlessly or snapping at people for no obvious reason? Do you feel weighed down by an overall sense of having little to offer yourself or anyone else?

If you've been suffering this kind of malaise with little or no relief, the mood repair strategies will probably be more effective with the guidance of a mental health professional. As well, you may benefit from antidepressant medication in combination with these strategies. There is some tentative evidence that a combination of medication and some of the more research-based mood repair strategies—such as cognitive restructuring in Chapter 4, behavioral activation in Chapter 5, and mindfulness meditation in Chapter 7—can be effective in treating major depression.

> **Recurrent or persistent thoughts of suicide are never to be ignored. If your mood state gets this low, call your mental health therapist or doctor immediately.**

The presence of suicidal thoughts or urges is another reason to seek professional help. People who are feeling moderate to severely depressed can get to the point where life seems hopeless and the future looks bleak; there seems to be no solution to life's problems except life's end. If you are having suicidal thoughts, especially if they have progressed to a plan or attempted suicide in the past, then you should definitely work with a mental health professional on your depression. The reason this is so important is that a therapist can monitor changes in your mood and suicide potential, and can ensure that measures are in place to keep you safe during times when your will to live may be especially low. In addition, some of the antidepressants can increase suicide risk, so it is especially important that your medication treatment is followed by a family physician or psychiatrist.

Many people who experience bouts of depression also struggle with drug or alcohol problems. This is understandable, since they may try to cope with difficult life circumstances by using substances to deal with the associated negative mood state. Alcohol in particular will actually worsen a depressed mood, however, and so using it (or any other substance) is not an effective response to feeling sad or distressed. Once again, it is advisable to work with a professional in efforts to break a habit of drug or alcohol abuse. You may find many of this book's mood repair strategies helpful in dealing with the mood fluctuations that can occur if you are trying to reduce or abstain from substance use. Nevertheless, mood repair on its own will be insufficient in treating substance abuse or dependence. Definitely consider contacting a drug and alcohol rehabilitation expert if you are struggling with a substance use problem.

As discussed in Chapter 1, some people struggle with repeated negative mood due to a major loss. The death of a spouse or child, a past physical or sexual trauma, and other major events are particularly toxic to mood. Suffering from posttraumatic stress disorder, or having recurring feelings of grief and sadness for years after the death of a loved one, may make it very difficult to do mood repair on your own and may require the help of a therapist. A therapist can help with the processing of negative emotion associated with a major past threat or loss. This type of therapeutic processing is very difficult to achieve on one's own.

Troubleshooting Your Mood Repair

At this point you may have tried some of the mood repair strategies, and I'm guessing you wouldn't have reached this point in the book if you hadn't gotten some benefit. But you may have been disappointed with the results in some cases and want to know what went wrong. Even though many of these strategies have been proven effective in down-regulating depressed mood, positive outcomes are never guaranteed, and results vary from person to person. Some strategies may not work for you at all, even though they work for others. Please don't give up, however! Instead, use the problem-solving strategy in Chapter 3 (Repair Strategy 10) to try to figure out why some (or most?) mood repair strategies have not worked for you.

> **Don't give up on mood repair before doing some troubleshooting to identify the problems.**

The following are some difficulties you may have encountered that could weaken your mood repair attempts.

MISMATCHES BETWEEN PROBLEMS AND MOOD REPAIR STRATEGIES

Have you been strategic in your approach to mood repair? Maybe you've focused on a mood repair strategy that is not a good match for the core problem that is driving your recurring depressed mood. For example, let's say you are feeling depressed because you are lonely, you have no friends, and you're cut off from your family. You decide to focus on depressive rumination, because you lose sleep brooding about how no one seems to like you. You spend time doing the exercises in Chapter 6, but you don't feel much better; although you do brood a bit less, you feel upset that you still have no friends. The main problems in this case are really your loneliness and social isolation, so you should be working on the strategies in Chapter 10. Those exercises would probably prove a lot more helpful for reducing your depression than the strategies in Chapter 6.

> **Aim mood repair at the *primary* cause(s) of your depressed mood.**

So, if your mood repair work is not helpful, reevaluate whether you've chosen the most effective strategy for the nature of your low mood. No one can be expected to use all of the mood repair strategies in this book; you should choose those that are most appropriate for your experience of depression.

> **TOOL FINDER** The strategies in Chapters 2 and 3 can help you pinpoint the causes and triggers of your lowered mood, so that you can target those in your mood repair work.

NEGATIVE EXPECTATIONS

Do negativity and skepticism dominate your thinking even when it comes to mood repair? You may be thinking, "OK, I'll give this a try, but I can't see it working for me." The problem with negative expectations is that they usually become self-fulfilling prophecies: If you don't think something will work, you may well put less effort into it, and because of less effort, the strategies may prove less effective. Be honest with yourself, and take a hard look at your expectations. If you think you've been suffering from cynicism and low expectations, use the exercises in Chapter 4 to challenge your preconceived ideas that might be undermining your efforts.

> Maintain realistic expectations about the benefits of mood repair.

DIFFICULTY ACCEPTING THE EMOTION REGULATION PERSPECTIVE

Are you having difficulty accepting the basic idea that we can take some control over our emotions? Even though Chapter 7 talks about accepting emotions and allowing them to flow more naturally, without prejudice or judgment, the intention of mindfulness meditation is that unwanted negative emotions will dissipate. There is never a suggestion that individuals should simply wallow in their own despair. This is a matter of *taking control by letting go.* Moreover, it is likely that you have been engaged in emotion regulation all your life, even if you did not label it as such. When people are feeling down or distressed, it is natural for them to try to do something to change the way they feel. So, rather than approaching emotion regulation as a foreign concept, think of this book as offering advice on how to change, expand, or revise your current mood repair efforts to increase their effectiveness.

> Accept emotion regulation as a key component of positive mental health.

INTENSE AND PROLONGED DEPRESSION

Have you struggled with depression for many years? If so, any changes in how you deal with the blues will take time to yield results. Also, your depression may meet diagnostic criteria for major depression or bipolar disorder—in which case you should be working with a mental health professional, as discussed earlier in this chapter. It is reasonable to expect that the longer you've been depressed, the more intense and interfering your depressed moods will be, and the more mood repair work will be

needed to achieve noticeable benefit. If, for example, we take the individuals introduced in Chapter 1, Joan (with her history of major depression) would probably require
more mood repair work than Sarah (who
had been relatively free of intense
depressed moods until she went through
the separation from her husband).

> **Prolonged, intense depression and/
> or major life events may complicate
> your mood repair efforts.**

SIGNIFICANT LIFE ADVERSITIES

Are you experiencing more sadness and depression in your life because of a major
life stressor or loss of a loved one? If so, it will take more systematic, time-intensive
emotional work to deal with the adverse effects caused by such significant life adversity. Again, a mental health consultation is recommended in such cases, as discussed
earlier. You may also find that dealing with the event itself has to take priority, and
that management of its emotional consequences becomes a secondary consideration,
at least for a time.

INCONSISTENT APPLICATION OF STRATEGIES

Have you been consistent in your mood repair work, or have you taken a smorgasbord
approach to harnessing your negativity? Maybe you've tried some of the exercises, but
your applications in daily living have been hit-and-miss. There is a saying that practice
makes perfect, and this applies to emotion regulation as much as it does to learning any
other skill. For example, the mood repair strategies in Chapter 4 for countering negative thoughts and self-criticism take repeated practice before people begin to notice a
difference. In using this approach in my clinical practice for 20 years, I've found that
one or two attempts at cognitive restructuring make no difference in people's level of
depression. However, when they practice correcting their negative automatic thoughts
in different situations over time, people start to get more proficient with the technique,
and it becomes a more automatic, natural way of coping with the negative thinking
that causes them to feel depressed. And other mood repair strategies, such as physical exercise, mindfulness meditation, and behavioral activation, require systematic,
repeated application in response to daily mood. So if mood repair is not working for
you, take a look at your efforts and determine whether you've been consistent.

TIME MANAGEMENT PROBLEMS

Are you making time in your day for mood repair? Many people feel crushed by the
demands of work, family, home, and other responsibilities. Daily living can get so

crowded with obligations that the last thing you feel you can do is add another respon-sibility. And yet it is likely that we all waste some time during our days. Think of it this way: If you are suffering from regular bouts of depressed mood, these bouts will signif-icantly reduce your productivity and efficient use of time. By introducing mood repair strategies and decreasing the amounts of time you spend in the blues, you may actually end up with more time rather than less. Mood repair is all about taking time to look after yourself. Time spent exercising, meditating, dealing with negative thoughts is actually "me time"; it's time well spent in "recharging your emotional batteries," so you can more efficiently meet all the other challenges in your life.

The Meaning-of-Life Question

In Chapter 9, I have discussed the importance of life goals and the key role that goal attainment plays in our daily experience of feeling happy or sad. As noted in that chap-ter, goals are based on personal life values. And this raises a really big question: What is the ultimate purpose and meaning of our lives?

Chapter 14 has presented Seligman's five elements of enhanced quality of life or well-being: positive emotion, engagement, meaning, accomplishment, and positive relationships.[1] As discussed there, frequent experiences with positive emotion, and engagement in highly absorbing activities, are critical to flourishing in this life. How-ever, the last three elements—meaning, accomplishment, and positive relationships—refer to life values. The pursuit of accomplishment (at least in the forms of material achievement and success) is emphasized in North American society, and the impor-tance of connectedness (i.e., of maintaining close and intimate relations with family and friends) has been discussed in Chapters 10 and 11. The one value that we have not yet considered is that of *meaning*, or the sense of belonging to and serving something bigger than yourself. The concept of *spirituality* probably captures best this notion of meaning. In their self-help book *Breaking Free from Depression*, Jesse Wright and Laura McCray define spirituality as encompassing these elements:

- Purpose of life
- Faith in a higher power or greater good
- Connection to life and others
- Sense of inner wholeness

Wright and McCray go on to discuss the research on spirituality and depression, which indicates that people who engage in spiritual activities experience lower rates of depression and suicide and report more hope, optimism, and positive emotions. As you reflect on your personal life values, what role does spirituality play in your approach to living? Are you missing out on an enriching part of the human experience that enhances life's value and meaning? You might want to consider how you can develop deeper connections with your spiritual side.

It is difficult to explain what is meant by *meaningful engagement* or *fulfillment*. Most of us, however, know of individuals who are highly committed to some cause that is greater than themselves. For example, I've known many scientists and academics who are highly committed to their research pursuits, to the point where the pursuit of knowledge is the driving force in their life. I've also met religious people, as well as political or social activists, who are highly committed to worthy humanitarian causes. What is striking is the enthusiasm and incredible dedication these individuals have for their causes. They feel that their missions are much bigger than themselves, and they are fully engaged in pursuing well-defined goals related to those missions. And in their passion, a vibrant and strong connection to life itself is evident. In citing Viktor Frankl, the great Austrian psychiatrist and Holocaust survivor, Wright and McCray note that meaning involves moving beyond a self-centered existence to acting responsibly in the world, appreciating life, striving for a worthwhile goal, facing adversities, and connecting in love and kindness with those around us. So here is a series of questions you can ask yourself in your search for meaning:

"What am I passionate about in this life?"

"Am I engaged in a cause that is bigger than I am?"

"How much of my daily living is self-centered?"

"Do I have a sense of belonging to a community?"

"Am I showing love and compassion toward others? Am I concerned about enriching my connections with family, friends, and loved ones? Can I express and receive love and kindness? To what extent am I truly interested in and care about the lives of other people? Am I more invested in others or in me?"

It's difficult to imagine being happy and fulfilled if you also believe that your life has no value or purpose. To be happy, you must believe you are alive for some purpose that is greater than simply consuming the air you breathe or the other resources of this earth. What are you alive for? Do you have a purpose and meaning in life that is greater than yourself? I would encourage you to pursue the big question—to discover your passion, your mission, your purpose in life. And when you do this, you will have a sure foundation on which to base your mood repair strategies when you feel sad, discouraged, or depressed.

> **What is your mission, your passion in this life?**

resources

The books, organizations, and websites listed below provide useful information about a variety of topics related to repairing negative mood or enhancing positive mood. Many of these resources were consulted in the preparation of this book. They provide more detailed instruction on specific treatment approaches to depression, worry, and insomnia, as well as more in-depth discussion of such mood repair strategies as mindfulness, behavioral activation, compassion-focused therapy, and exercise. In addition, I have included a few books and websites on how to increase happiness and well-being in your life.

Books on Treating Depression

Addis, M. E., & Martell, C. R. (2004). *Overcoming depression one step at a time: The new behavioral activation approach to getting your life back*. Oakland, CA: New Harbinger.

Bieling, P. J., & Antony, M. M. (2003). *Ending the depression cycle: A step-by-step guide for preventing relapse*. Oakland, CA: New Harbinger.

Bonanno, G. A. (2009). *The other side of sadness: What the new science of bereavement tells us about life after loss*. New York: Basic Books.

Corcoran, J. (2009). *The depression solutions workbook*. Oakland, CA: New Harbinger.

Greenberger, D., & Padesky, C. A. (1995). *Mind over mood: A cognitive therapy treatment manual for clients*. New York: Guilford Press.

Ilardi, S. S. (2009). *The depression cure: The 6-step program to beat depression without drugs*. Cambridge, MA: Da Capo Press.

Leahy, R. L. (2010). *Beat the blues before they beat you: How to overcome depression*. Carlsbad, CA: Hay House.

Pettit, J. W., & Joiner, T. E. (2005). *The interpersonal solution to depression: A workbook for changing how you feel by changing how you relate*. Oakland, CA: New Harbinger.

Wright, J. H., & McCray, L. W. (2012). *Breaking free from depression: Pathways to wellness*. New York: Guilford Press.

Books on Treating Worry

Butler, G., & Hope, T. (2007). *Managing your mind: The mental fitness guide*. Oxford: Oxford University Press.

Clark, D. A., & Beck, A. T. (2012). *The anxiety and worry workbook: The cognitive behavioral solution.* New York: Guilford Press.

Leahy, R. L. (2005). *The worry cure: Seven steps to stop worry from stopping you.* New York: Harmony Books.

McKay, M., Davis, M., & Fanning, P. (2011). *Thoughts and feelings* (4th ed.). Oakland, CA: New Harbinger.

Meares, K., & Freeston, M. (2008). *Overcoming worry: A self-help guide using cognitive behavioural techniques.* London: Constable & Robinson.

Books on Mindfulness and Compassion

Germer, C. K. (2009). *The mindful path to self-compassion: Freeing yourself from destructive thoughts and emotions.* New York: Guilford Press.

Gilbert, P. (2009). *The compassionate mind: A new approach to life's challenges.* Oakland, CA: New Harbinger.

Hanson, R., with Mendius, R. (2009). *Buddha's brain: The practical neuroscience of happiness, love, and wisdom.* Oakland, CA: New Harbinger.

Kabat-Zinn, J. (2005). *Full catastrophe living: Using the wisdom of your body and mind to face stress, pain, and illness.* New York: Delta.

McQuaid, J. R., & Carmona, P. E. (2004). *Peaceful mind.* Oakland, CA: New Harbinger.

Strosahl, K. D., & Robinson, P. J. (2008). *The mindfulness and acceptance workbook for depression: Using acceptance and commitment therapy to move through depression and create a life worth living.* Oakland, CA: New Harbinger.

Teasdale, J. D., Williams, J. M. G., & Segal, Z. V. (2014). *The mindful way workbook: An 8-week program to free yourself from depression and emotional distress.* New York: Guilford Press.

Williams, M., Teasdale, J., Segal, Z., & Kabat-Zinn, J. (2007). *The mindful way through depression: Freeing yourself from chronic unhappiness.* New York: Guilford Press.

Books on Exercise, Insomnia, and Expressing Emotion

Edinger, J. D., & Carney, C. E. (2008). *Overcoming insomnia: A cognitive-behavioral therapy approach workbook.* Oxford: Oxford University Press.

Otto, M. W., & Smits, J. A. J. (2011). *Exercise for mood and anxiety: Proven strategies for overcoming depression and enhancing well-being.* New York: Oxford University Press.

Pennebaker, J. W. (1997). *Opening up: The healing power of expressing emotion* (rev. ed.). New York: Guilford Press.

Silberman, S. A. (2008). *The insomnia workbook.* Oakland, CA: New Harbinger.

Books on Happiness and Well-Being

Ehrenreich, B. (2009). *Bright-sided: How the relentless promotion of positive thinking has undermined America.* New York: Metropolitan Books/Holt.

Lyubomirsky, S. (2008). *The how of happiness: A new approach to getting the life you want.* New York: Penguin.

Seligman, M. E. P. (2011). *Flourish: A visionary new understanding of happiness and well-being.* New York: Free Press.

Informative Organizations

Association for Behavioral and Cognitive Therapies (ABCT)
305 Seventh Avenue, 16th Floor
New York, NY 10001-6008, USA
Phone: 1-212-647-1890
Fax: 1-212-647-1865
Website: *www.abct.org*

Academy of Cognitive Therapy (ACT)
260 South Broad Street, 18th Floor
Philadelphia, PA 19102, USA
Phone: 1-267-350-7683
Fax: 1-215-731-2182
E-mail: *info@academyofct.org*
Website: *www.academyofct.org*

Australian Association for Cognitive and Behaviour Therapy (AACBT)
P.O. Box 4040
Nowra East, New South Wales 2541, Australia
Fax: 07 3041 0415
E-mail: *info@aacbt.org*
Website: *www.aacbt.org*

British Association for Behavioural and Cognitive Psychotherapies (BABCP)
Imperial House
Hornby Street
Bury, Lancashire BL9 5BN, United Kingdom
Phone: 0161 705 4304
Fax: 0161 705 4306
E-mail: *babcp@babcp.com*
Website: *www.babcp.com*

Canadian Psychological Association (CPA)
141 Laurier Avenue West, Suite 702
Ottawa, Ontario K1P 5J3, Canada
Phone: 1-888-472-0657 (toll-free in Canada) or 1-613-237-2144
Fax: 613-237-1674
E-mail: *cpa@cpa.ca*
Website: *www.cpa.ca*

Helpful Websites

For information on the following topics, see these websites:

Happiness and well-being
> *www.authentichappiness.sas.upenn.edu*
> *www.actionforhappiness.org*

Dieting
> *www.beckdietsolution.com*

Exercise
> *www.crossfit.com*
> *www.fitness.com*
> *www.fitness.gov*

Relaxation and breathing instructions
> *www.mindtools.com*

Mental health and fitness
> *www.nice.org.uk*
> *www.cmha.ca/mental_health/mental-fitness-tips*

Depression
> *www.bluepages.anu.edu.au*
> *www.nimh.nih.gov/health/topics/depression*

Self-help treatment for depression
> *www.moodgym.anu.edu.au*
> *www.moodjuice.scot.nhs.uk/depression.asp*
> *www.helpguide.org/mental/depression_tips.htm*

references

Chapter 1

1. Howland, R. H., Schettler, P. J., Rapoport, M. H., Mischoulon, D., Schneider, T., Fasiczka, A., et al. (2008). Clinical features and functioning of patients with minor depression. *Psychotherapy and Psychosomatics, 77*, 384–389.

2. Bonanno, G. A., Goorin, L., & Coifman, K. G. (2008). Sadness and grief. In M. Lewis, J. M. Haviland-Jones, & L. F. Barrett (Eds.), *Handbook of emotions* (3rd ed., pp. 797–810). New York: Guilford Press.

3. Chepenik, L. G., Cornew, L. A., & Farah, M. J. (2007). The influence of sad mood on cognition. *Emotion, 7*, 802–811. [See the introduction to this paper for a review of the topic.]

4. Ito, T. A., & Cacioppo, J. T. (2005). Variations on a human universal: Individual differences in positivity offset and negativity bias. *Cognition and Emotion, 19*, 1–26.

5. Kessler, R. C., Berglund, P., Demler, O., Jin, R., Koretz, D., Merikangas, K. R., et al. (2003). The epidemiology of major depressive disorder: Results from the National Comorbidity Survey Replication (NCS-R). *Journal of the American Medical Association, 289*, 3095–3105.

6. Kessler, R. C., Zhao, S., Blazer, D. G., & Swartz, M. (1997). Prevalence, correlates, and course of minor depression and major depression in the National Comorbidity Survey. *Journal of Affective Disorders, 45*, 19–30.

7. Meeks, T. W., Vahia, I. V., Lavretsky, H., Kulkarni, G., & Jeste, D. V. (2011). A tune in "A minor" and "B major": A review of epidemiology, illness course, and public health implications of subthreshold depression in older adults. *Journal of Affective Disorders, 129*, 126–142.

8. Werner, K., & Gross, J. J. (2010). Emotion regulation and psychopathology: A conceptual framework. In A. M. Kring & D. M. Sloan (Eds.), *Emotion regulation and psychopathology: A transdiagnostic approach to etiology and treatment* (pp. 13–37). New York: Guilford Press.

9. Fairholme, C. P., Boisseau, C. L., Ellard, K. K., Ehrenreich, J. T., & Barlow, D. H. (2010). Emotions, emotion regulation, and psychological treatment: A unified perspective. In A. M. Kring & D. M. Sloan (Eds.), *Emotion regulation and psychopathology: A transdiagnostic approach to etiology and treatment* (pp. 283–309). New York: Guilford Press.

10. Corcoran, K. M., Farb, N., Anderson, A., & Segal, Z. V. (2010). Mindfulness and emotion regulation: Outcomes and possible mediating mechanisms. In A. M. Kring & D. M. Sloan (Eds.), *Emotion regulation and psychopathology: A transdiagnostic approach to etiology and treatment* (pp. 339–355). New York: Guilford Press.

11. Fredrickson, B. L., & Losada, M. F. (2005). Positive affect and the complex dynamics of human flourishing. *American Psychologist, 60,* 678–686.

12. Seligman, M. E. P. (2011). *Flourish: A visionary new understanding of happiness and well-being.* New York: Free Press.

Chapter 2

1. U.S. Mood (Weekly). Retrieved on July 16, 2012, from *www.gallup.com/poll/151166/Mood-Weekly. aspx*

2. Carstensen, L. L., Pasupathi, M., Mayr, U., & Nesselroade, J. R. (2000). Emotional experience in everyday life across the adult life span. *Journal of Personality and Social Psychology, 79,* 644–655.

3. Golder, S. A., & Macy, M. M. (2011). Diurnal and seasonal mood vary with work, sleep, and day-length across diverse cultures. *Science, 333,* 1878–1881.

4. Dodds, P. S., Harris, K. D., Kloumann, I. M., Bliss, C. A., & Danforth, C. M. (2011). Temporal patterns of happiness and information in a global social network: Hedonometrics and Twitter. *PLoS One, 6*(12), e26752, 1–25.

Chapter 3

1. Kahneman, D., Krueger, A. B., Schkade, D. A., Schwarz, N., & Stone, A. A. (2004). A survey method for characterizing daily life experience: The Day Reconstruction Method. *Science, 306,* 1776–1780.

Chapter 5

1. Martell, C. R., Addis, M. E., & Jacobson, N. S. (2001). *Depression in context: Strategies for guided action.* New York: Norton.

Chapter 6

1. Nolen-Hoeksema, S., Wisco, B. E., & Lyubomirsky, S. (2008). Rethinking rumination. *Perspectives on Psychological Science, 3,* 400–424.

2. Papageorgiou, C., & Wells, A. (2004). Nature, functions, and beliefs about depressive rumination. In C. Papageorgiou & A. Wells (Eds.), *Depressive rumination: Nature, theory and treatment* (pp. 3–20). Chichester, UK: Wiley.

3. Wisco, B. E., & Nolen-Hoeksema, S. (2008). Ruminative response style. In K. S. Dobson & D. J. A. Dozois (Eds.), *Risk factors in depression* (pp. 221–236). Amsterdam: Elsevier.

4. Treynor, W., Gonzalez, R., & Nolen-Hoeksema, S. (2003). Rumination reconsidered: A psychometric analysis. *Cognitive Therapy and Research, 27,* 247–259.

Chapter 7

1. Segal, Z. V., Bieling, P., Young, T., MacQueen, G., Cooke, R., Martin, L., et al. (2010). Antidepressant monotherapy vs sequential pharmacotherapy and mindfulness-based cognitive therapy, or placebo, for relapse prophylaxis in recurrent depression. *Archives of General Psychiatry, 67,* 1256–1264.
2. Bieling, P. J., Hawley, L. L., Bloch, R. T., Corcoran, K. M., Levitan, R. D., Young, L. T., et al. (2012). Treatment-specific changes in decentering following mindfulness-based cognitive therapy versus antidepressant medication or placebo for prevention of depressive relapse. *Journal of Consulting and Clinical Psychology, 80,* 365–372.
3. Bylsma, L. M., Morris, B. H., & Rottenberg, J. (2008). A meta-analysis of emotional reactivity in major depressive disorder. *Clinical Psychology Review, 28,* 676–691.
4. Maltby, J., Lewis, C. A., Freeman, A., Day, L., Cruise, S. M., & Breslin, M. J. (2010). Religion and health: The application of a cognitive-behavioural framework. *Mental Health, Religion and Culture, 13,* 749–759.

Chapter 8

1. Williams, J. M. G., Barnhofer, T., Hermans, D., Raes, F., Crane, C., Watkins, E., et al. (2007). Autobiographical memory specificity and emotional disorders. *Psychological Bulletin, 133,* 122–148.
2. Joormann, J., Siemer, M., & Gotlib, I. H. (2007). Mood regulation in depression: Differential effects of distraction and recall of happy memories on sad mood. *Journal of Abnormal Psychology, 116,* 484–490.
3. Holmes, E. A., Lang, T. J., & Shah, D. M. (2009). Developing interpretation bias modification as a "cognitive vaccine" for depressed mood: Imaging positive events makes you feel better than thinking about them verbally. *Journal of Abnormal Psychology, 118,* 76–88.
4. Dalgleish, T., & Yiend, J. (2006). The effects of suppressing a negative autobiographical memory on concurrent intrusions and subsequent autobiographical recall in dysphoria. *Journal of Abnormal Psychology, 115,* 467–473.

Chapter 9

1. Snyder, C. R. (2002). Hope theory: Rainbows in the mind. *Psychological Inquiry, 13,* 249–275.
2. Stone, A. A., Schwartz, J. E., Schwartz, N., Schkade, D., Krueger, A., & Kahneman, D. (2006). A population approach to the study of emotion: Diurnal rhythms of a working day examined with the day reconstruction method. *Emotion, 6,* 139–149.
3. Holmes, E. A., & Mathews, A. (2010). Mental imagery in emotion and emotional disorders. *Clinical Psychology Review, 30,* 349–362.
4. Kappes, H. B., Oettingen, G., Mayer, D., & Maglio, S. (2011). Sad mood promotes self-initiated mental contrasting of future and reality. *Emotion, 11,* 1206–1222.

Chapter 10

1. Timmons, K. A., & Joiner, T. E. (2008). Reassurance seeking and negative feedback seeking. In K. S. Dobson & D. J. A. Dozois (Eds.), *Risk factors in depression* (pp. 429–446). Amsterdam: Elsevier.
2. Weissman, M. M., Markowitz, J. C., & Klerman, G. L. (2000). *Comprehensive guide to interpersonal psychotherapy.* New York: Basic Books.

Chapter 11

1. Gilbert, P. (2009). *The compassionate mind: A new approach to life's challenges.* Oakland, CA: New Harbinger.
2. Neff, K. D. (2003). The development and validation of a scale to measure self-compassion. *Self and Identity, 2,* 223–250.
3. Otake, K., Shimai, S., Tanaka-Matsumi, J., Otsui, K., & Fredrickson, B. L. (2006). Happy people become happier through kindness: A counting kindnesses intervention. *Journal of Happiness Studies, 7,* 361–375.
4. Papa, A., & Bonanno, G. A. (2008). Smiling in the face of adversity: The interpersonal and intrapersonal functions of smiling. *Emotion, 8,* 1–12.
5. Erickson, T. M., & Abelson, J. L. (2012). Even the downhearted may be uplifted: Moral evaluation in the daily life of clinically depressed and anxious adults. *Journal of Social and Clinical Psychology, 31,* 707–728.
6. Leary, M. R., Tate, E. B., Adams, C. E., Allen, A. B., & Hancock, J. (2007). Self-compassion and reactions to unpleasant self-relevant events: The implications of treating oneself kindly. *Journal of Personality and Social Psychology, 92,* 887–904.

Chapter 12

1. Otto, M. W., & Smits, J. A. J. (2011). *Exercise for mood and anxiety: Proven strategies for overcoming depression and enhancing well-being.* New York: Oxford University Press.
2. Conn, V. S. (2010). Depressive symptom outcomes of physical activity interventions: Meta-analysis findings. *Annals of Behavioral Medicine, 39,* 128–138.
3. Stathopoulou, G., Powers, M. B., Berry, A. C., Smits, J. A. J., & Otto, M. W. (2006). Exercise interventions for mental health: A quantitative and qualitative review. *Clinical Psychology: Science and Practice, 13,* 179–193.
4. De Mello, M. T., de Aquino Lemos, V., Antunes, H. K. M., Bittencourt, L., Santos-Silva, R., & Tufik, S. (2013). Relationship between physical activity and depression and anxiety symptoms: A population study. *Journal of Affective Disorders, 149,* 241–246.
5. World Health Organization. (2011). *Global recommendations on physical activity for health: 18-64 year old.* Retrieved April 12, 2013, from *www.who.int/dietphysicalactivity/physical-activity-recommendations-18-64years.pdf*

6. U.S. Department of Health and Human Services. (2008). *2008 physical activity guidelines for Americans.* Retrieved April 12, 2013, from *www.health.gov/paguidelines/guidelines/summary.aspx*
7. Centers for Disease Control and Prevention. (2011). Unhealthy sleep-related behaviors—12 states, 2009. *Morbidity and Mortality Weekly Reports, 60,* 233–242. Retrieved April 16, 2013, from *www.cdc.gov/mmwr/PDF/wk/mm6008.pdf*
8. Silberman, S. A. (2008). *The insomnia workbook.* Oakland, CA: New Harbinger.
9. Sanchez-Villegas, A., Delgado-Rodriguez, M., Alonso, A., Schlatter, J., Lahortiga, F., Serra Majem, L., et al. (2009). Association of the Mediterranean dietary pattern with the incidence of depression. *Archives of General Psychiatry, 66,* 1090–1098.

Chapter 13

1. Martell, C. R., Addis, M. E., & Jacobson, N. S. (2001). *Depression in context: Strategies for guided action.* New York: Norton.
2. Steel, P. (2007). The nature of procrastination: A meta-analytic and theoretical review of quintessential self-regulatory failure. *Psychological Bulletin, 133,* 65–94.

Chapter 14

1. Layard, P. R. G. (2011). *Happiness: Lessons from a new science* (2nd ed.). London: Penguin Books.
2. Seligman, M. E. P. (2011). *Flourish: A visionary new understanding of happiness and well-being.* New York: Free Press.
3. Lyubomirsky, S., King, L., & Diener, E. (2005). The benefits of frequent positive affect: Does happiness lead to success? *Psychological Bulletin, 131,* 803–855.
4. Emmons, R. A., & McCullough, M. E. (2003). Counting blessings versus burdens: An experimental investigation of gratitude and subjective well-being in daily life. *Journal of Personality and Social Psychology, 84,* 377–389.
5. Lambert, N. M., Fincham, F. D., & Stillman, T. F. (2012). Gratitude and depressive symptoms: The role of positive reframing and positive emotion. *Cognition and Emotion, 26,* 615–633.
6. Fredrickson, B. L., & Losada, M. F. (2005). Positive affect and the complex dynamics of human flourishing. *American Psychologist, 60,* 678–686.
7. Schwartz, R. M. (1997). Consider the simple screw: Cognitive science, quality improvement, and psychotherapy. *Journal of Consulting and Clinical Psychology, 65,* 970–983.
8. Simon, H. A. (1956). Rational choice and the structure of the environment. *Psychological Review, 63,* 129–138.
9. Schwartz, B., Ward, A., Monterosso, J., Lyubomirsky, S., White, K., & Lehman, D. R. (2002). Maximizing versus satisficing: Happiness is a matter of choice. *Journal of Personality and Social Psychology, 83,* 1178–1197.
10. Gable, S. L., Gonzaga, G. C., & Strachman, A. (2006). Will you be there for me when things go

right?: Supportive responses to positive event disclosures. *Journal of Personality and Social Psychology, 91*, 904–917.

Chapter 15

1. Seligman, M. E. P. (2011). *Flourish: A visionary new understanding of happiness and well-being.* New York: Free Press.

index

about the author

David A. Clark, PhD, is Professor of Psychology at the University of New Brunswick, Canada, where he also has had a private practice for 25 years. Dr. Clark is a widely recognized authority on cognitive behavior therapy for anxiety and depression and is the author of numerous books, including *The Anxiety and Worry Workbook* (with Aaron T. Beck) and *Overcoming Obsessive Thoughts* (with Christine Purdon). He is a Founding Fellow of the Academy of Cognitive Therapy and a Fellow of the Canadian Psychological Association.